VAGUS NERVE

Activate Your Vagus Nerve
with Stimulation and Practical Exercises
to Reduce Anxiety, Depression,
Chronic Illness, Inflammation, PTSD,
Autoimmune Disease, Fibromyalgia
and Much More

Matthew Pain

© Copyright 2019 by Matthew Pain - All rights reserved.

This Book is provided with the sole purpose of providing relevant information on a specific topic for which every reasonable effort has been made to ensure that it is both accurate and reasonable. Nevertheless, by purchasing this Book, you consent to the fact that the author, as well as the publisher, are in no way experts on the topics contained herein, regardless of any claims as such that may be made within. As such, any suggestions or recommendations that are made within are done so purely for entertainment value. It is recommended that you always consult a professional prior to undertaking any of the advice or techniques discussed within.

This is a legally binding declaration that is considered both valid and fair by both the Committee of Publishers Association and the American Bar Association and should be considered as legally binding within the United States.

The reproduction, transmission, and duplication of any of the content found herein, including any specific or extended information, will be done as an illegal act regardless of the end form the information ultimately takes. This includes copied versions of the work, both physical, digital, and audio unless the express consent of the Publisher is provided beforehand. Any additional rights reserved.

Furthermore, the information that can be found within the pages described forthwith shall be considered both accurate and truthful when it comes to the recounting of facts. As such, any use, correct or incorrect, of the provided information will render the Publisher free of responsibility as to the actions taken outside of their direct purview. Regardless, there are zero scenarios where the original author or the Publisher can be deemed liable in any fashion for any damages or hardships that may result from any of the information discussed herein.

Additionally, the information in the following pages is intended only for informational purposes and should thus be thought of as universal. As befitting its nature, it is presented without assurance regarding its prolonged validity or interim quality. Trademarks that are mentioned are done without written consent and can in no way be considered an endorsement from the trademark holder.

CONTENTS

Introduction..5

Part I - The Vagus Nerve..9
Chapter 1: What is the Vagus Nerve?........................11
Chapter 2: Importance of the Vagus Nerve...............19
Chapter 3: History of the Vagus Nerve......................25
Chapter 4: The Vagus Nerve and the Nervous System.............31
Chapter 5: The Vagus Nerve and the Body................41
Chapter 6: The Vagus Nerve and the Mind................49

Part II - Pathologies of the Vagus Nerve....................57
Chapter 7: The Vagus Nerve and Anxiety..................59
Chapter 8: The Vagus Nerve and Depression............67
Chapter 9: The Vagus Nerve and Chronic Illness......75
Chapter 10: The Vagus Nerve and Inflammation......85
Chapter 11: The Vagus Nerve and PTSD....................93
Chapter 12: The Vagus Nerve and Autoimmune Disease.........101
Chapter 13: The Vagus Nerve and Fibromyalgia......111
Chapter 14: The Vagus Nerve and Sleep Disorders...............117
Chapter 15: The Vagus Nerve and Epilepsy..............125
Chapter 16: The Vagus Nerve and Rheumatoid Arthritis........131
Chapter 17: The Vagus Nerve and Other Symptoms...............137

Part III - Therapies and Exercises for Stimulating the Vagus Nerve..143
Chapter 18: Vagus Nerve Stimulation......................145
Chapter 19: Breathing to Stimulate the Vagus Nerve.............151
Chapter 20: Temperature to Stimulate the Vagus Nerve........157
Chapter 21: Singing to Stimulate the Vagus Nerve...............161
Chapter 22: Coffee Enema to Stimulate the Vagus Nerve......165
Chapter 23: Mindfulness to Stimulate the Vagus Nerve........171
Chapter 24: Movement to Stimulate the Vagus Nerve..........177

Chapter 25: Balancing the Gut Microbiome to Heal the Vagus Nerve...181
Conclusion..187

Introduction

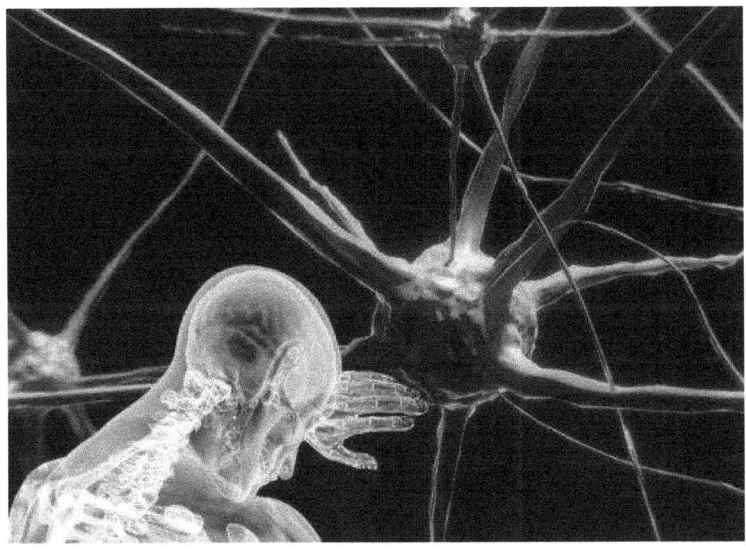

Have you ever had that moment in life where you stop and are hit with the sudden realization of just how *insane* it is that your entire body is capable of regulating itself? You cannot will yourself to stop breathing or for your heart to stop—even if you try your hardest, there is no possible way for you to manage to override those life-giving processes that keep you alive. Sure, you can hold your breath, but you are going to pass out long before you suffocate yourself. This is because of your autonomic nervous system—a series of nerves within your body that keep you alive. They regulate everything from your heartbeat to your ability to digest food. They control your breathing and ability to manage all of the muscles in your body that are responsible for keeping you alive.

Essentially, your automatic nervous system is responsible for keeping you alive—and it does so entirely unconsciously. You are never aware of the processes in your brain that are actively keeping your heart regulated or your diaphragm moving in regular intervals to keep you alive. Within this automatic nervous system, the brain is connected to the rest of the body, to all of those important parts that keep your body alive and functioning with impressive ease, through what is known as the vagus nerve.

The vagus nerve, simplified down, is a circuit of nerve cells that root throughout the body and brain—they go down to the body, interacting with the heart, lungs, and abdomen, and return back to the brain. This has one simple function—it allows the brain to communicate with those crucial parts. However, sometimes, that nerve circuit can malfunction, and when it does, there can be significant impacts on the individual. Just as how a car that has a dysfunctional electrical system may struggle to run effectively, the human body struggles when there are any errors in the vagus nerves.

This book will open your eyes to the myriad of ways that the vagus nerve can directly and negatively impact your life. It is so intrinsically involved in the body's structure that it has even been found to be relevant to treating PTSD, epilepsy, and even rheumatoid arthritis. You will be introduced to the importance of the nerve itself before seeing several of the pathologies related to the vagus nerve. Lastly, you will be introduced to several techniques that you can use to stimulate your vagus nerve—in stimulating the vagus nerve, you are able to sort of reset it, allowing yourself to give it the jump-start it needs in order to start working effectively so it can start regulating your body exactly as it was intended to.

As you read through this book, you will learn all of the information that you will need in order to regulate your own vagus nerve with ease—while there are treatments out there that will literally stimulate the vagus nerve for you when implanted, there are also ways that you can essentially trigger your body to regulate it yourself. Ranging from deep breathing to yoga, there are a wide range of ways that you can regulate that nerve, and in doing so, you can find relief.

Part I
The Vagus Nerve

Chapter 1: What is the Vagus Nerve?

Everything about you is regulated by nerves. From your very thoughts to the way you move your body and what keeps you alive, everything is related to your nerves. Your nerves are the very wiring that allows you to exist and function. They are the wiring that connects the body to the mind and they run throughout the whole body. They are different sizes, all running to different areas, and allowing your entire body to interact as once integrated being, one complete system that is entirely able to work together effectively and cohesively.

Nerves themselves come in two distinct forms, based on origin— there are spinal nerves, which connect the spinal cord to the rest of the body, and there are cranial nerves, which connect the body to the brain. There are 13 different cranial nerves within the body, existing in pairs that connect to both hemispheres of the brain. These nerves are responsible for a wide range of information being transferred quickly and efficiently to the brain.

Nerves

Nerves themselves are cells that allow for electrochemical nerve impulses to travel throughout the body. These impulses, known as action potentials, are how the nerves communicate with each other. When you touch or otherwise interact with something, nerves have activated that trigger and send those same action potentials back throughout the nervous system and all the way to the brain, where they are then processed and treated accordingly.

These nerves are formed by an axon, which processes the impulse, and the sheathing around it. The nerves are said to *innervate*, or provide information and control, certain parts of the body. When an area is innervated by a specific nerve, that means that the particular nerve being discussed is responsible for the sensory movement and information at that spot.
When you speak about nerves, sometimes they directly interact with the same side of the body, known as ipsilateral, or the other side of the body, known as contralateral.

Your nerves are designed to carry impulses and action potentials almost instantaneously—they may trigger immediately and some of the fastest nerves are able to process at a speed of 120 m/s, during which the impulse is constantly being translated from an electrical impulse into a chemical impulse at the end of the axon, where chemicals are then released that interact with the next nerve in line in the sequence, where the nerve is then triggered, cuing it to create another electrical impulse. Basically, your nerves are constantly translating the sensory information that is going from the brain to your body, or from your body to your brain, in a constant loop from chemical to electrical to chemical again.

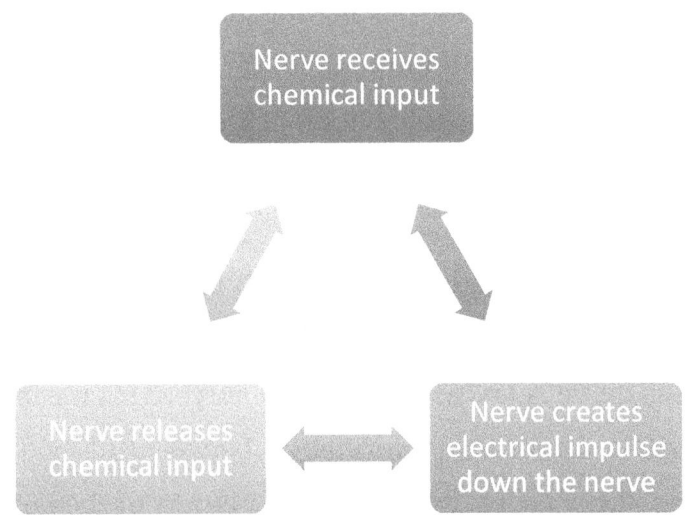

The Vagus Nerve

Longer than any other nerve in your autonomic nervous system, the vagus nerve wanders through the body. In fact, that is where it got its name—the name "vagus" comes directly from the Latin word for wandering. The nerve itself wanders through the body, allowing it to function normally when all is well with it. It regulates your body, allowing you to literally survive.

Initially, the vagus nerve was known as the pneumogastric nerve—pneumo referring to the lungs while gastric refers to the stomach. It is the tenth cranial nerve, sometimes written as CN

X. It is the primary interface between the parasympathetic nervous system and the brain, meaning it is what allows the brain to control much of the parasympathetic system without your conscious awareness. Despite the fact that the nerve comes in pairs and you have two of them, it is largely referred to just as the one vagus nerve—do not be fooled, however; there are two of them.

There are nerves throughout your entire body—these nerves are controlling everything about you. One such nerve is the vagus nerve. This nerve is known as a cranial nerve. This means that it is involved in translating information between the body to the brain. The vagus nerve, in particular, is a part of the autonomic nervous system—this is the system of nerves that is largely unconsciously controlled. It, then, is largely responsible for unconscious actions of the body.

The nerve itself directly interacts with several parts of the body, namely the heart, lungs, and digestive tract. This makes the vagus nerve so incredibly important—it is involved in regulating the heart, breathing, and digestion. Without it, your body would not be able to regulate these functions.

Purpose of the Vagus Nerve

The vagus nerve has several different purposes, but at its simplest, it is afferent—this means that it receives input from the senses and travels back to the brain. It is meant to be constantly regulating the body based on sensory stimuli, at its simplest. In particular, there are four key functions of this particular cranial nerve. These four functions are receiving sensory information for the following:

- **Sensory Input:** Receives information from the heart, the lungs, the throat, and the abdomen

- **Taste Input:** Provides the sensation of tasting

- **Motor:** Provides the function of movement within the muscles that are necessary and responsible for swallowing and speaking

- **Parasympathetic nervous system:** Regulates the function of digestion, breathing, and the heart rate

Those four functions, however, can be divided into seven even more specific functions. Within these seven functions, the vagus nerve is able to regulate a significant portion of the human body. These functions include:

- **Regulating the sympathetic nervous system:** It allows for the control and regulation of alertness, the circulatory system, and respiration. The vagus nerve will directly allow for the brain to regulate this system, allowing for a state of alertness and feeling of high energy. The activation of the sympathetic nervous system creates the fight-flight-freeze response.

- **Regulating the parasympathetic nervous system:** In contrast, it also allows for the regulation of the parasympathetic system. This system decreases the alertness one feels, instead of triggering relaxation and digestion. The activation of the parasympathetic nervous system triggers the rest-and-digest state.

- **Facilitating communication from the brain and the gut:** The vagus nerve creates the route that allows information to be transferred from the guts and digestive system all the way back to the brain.

- **Allowing and triggering a state of relaxation:** Along with the activation of the parasympathetic nervous system, the vagus nerve triggers the diaphragm to slow, creating the effect of deeper breathing, allowing for further relaxation.

- **Anti-inflammatory:** The vagus nerve is able to send out signals to the rest of the body that trigger an anti-inflammatory message to be received, allowing for inflammation levels to decrease.

- **Regulating both one's heart rate and blood pressure:** The vagus nerve is directly responsible for heart regulation and blood pressure. When it does not activate properly, it can lead to issues, such as the loss of consciousness or blood pressure to grow too high.

- **Managing and regulating fear and anxiety:** Because the vagus nerve regulates the sympathetic and parasympathetic nervous systems, it is able to tell the body when fear is appropriate, and when it is time to calm down and regulate that fear.

Chapter 2: Importance of the Vagus Nerve

Considering it is in charge of some of the most important functions within your body, namely regulating your ability to have a beating heart and breathe, it becomes incredibly apparent that your vagus nerve is incredibly important. In fact, it is believed to be one of the most important nerves within the body. Without it, or with it completely dysfunctional, a normal existence would be nearly impossible. Because of the fact that it is so crucial to so many of these important functions to survive, it has garnered plenty of attention in recent days.

Without the vagus nerve, you will be unable to do anything. You could not digest your food. You could not breathe when you slept. Your heart would stop beating. You would cease to live. The vagus nerve, when dysfunctional, disrupts nearly every major function in some way—it can lead to heart irregularities, breathing irregularities, digestive problems, and more, all because without this simple nerve pair, the brain cannot regulate it. Largely speaking, the importance of the vagus nerve lies in the fact that it is directly influential to the regulation of the autonomic nervous system.

This nerve becomes incredibly crucial to understand for one crucial reason—you can regulate it with ease. You can use the vagus nerve, learning how to stimulate it when necessary to regulate your own body. The nerve is there, just waiting for you to truly utilize it, and if you do, you are able to regulate the response of it simply by knowing how to regulate yourself.

The Mind-Body Connection

The mind and body are closely interrelated—two sides to the same coin, and yet, they cannot fully communicate without help. The nerves, namely the vagus nerve, communicates between the two, creating the conduit through which the nerve impulses are translated and passed along to enable the body to communicate with the brain. Without these impulses, the nervous system cannot get the regulation it needs. The mind cannot regulate the body if it does not receive feedback from the body. Think of the entire human body as a computer for a moment—the brain is like the processor while the rest of the body is every source through which the processor receives information to allow it to create outputs. Without the keyboard, the mouse, or the touchscreen, you cannot interact with the processor, and without being able to interact with the processor, you cannot expect anything to happen. The screen will not pull up that cat video or do the math on the calculator that you want to happen simply because there is no input going on.

The vagus nerve allows for that input, and then it allows you to regulate the body as well. Because the vagus nerve is so closely related to awareness and keeping the human body alive and processing, it is crucial to human survival.

The Vagus Nerve and Emotional Regulation

Another crucial factor of the vagus nerve is the fact that it is directly responsible for your ability to self-regulate. It is what calms you when you are stressed. When you meditate or do yoga to relax or calm yourself, you are unknowingly activating your vagus nerve. That stimulation creates the calming effect that you are feeling.

While it may seem counterproductive to see someone saying that stimulation is what is regulating them, that is exactly what you will see when you understand the vagus nerve. Stimulating it, which can happen in several different methods, can trigger that ability toward emotional regulation. You can calm yourself down, triggering yourself to tear yourself from the sympathetic fight-flight-freeze response over to the parasympathetic rest-and-digest mode. This, then, allows you plenty of options on its own—think about what that implication is. You can essentially, through understanding biology, hijack your gut reaction, that tendency toward fight-flight-freeze, and allow yourself to instead calm down.

That emotional regulation is powerful. It means that people can take control of their emotional states with a deep breathing exercise or some other method that will allow for a trigger and stimulation of the vagus nerve. When you learn this process, you give yourself another coping mechanism, a way to relieve your suffering and take your own mental wellness into your own hands. If you are afraid? You are able to activate your vagus nerve to help. Suffering from PTSD? Your vagus nerve can help with that, too. Several issues can be managed relatively simply, all through learning to take control of your vagus nerve.

Of course, it is important to remember that this book, while intended to be a guide to regulating your health and several issues through triggering your vagus nerve, is not meant to substitute seeing a doctor. This book does not, in any way, recommend you should overrule what your doctor has deemed as the best treatment of yourself. You should always take the advice of medical professionals, as they know exactly what is happening with your own body. They are able to look at you, interact with you, and create customized treatment plans and diagnoses that this book is not qualified to make. Please do not stop any treatment regimens you are currently undergoing in lieu of the advice provided within this book without first speaking to your doctor.

Activating the Vagus Nerve

Understanding that you can use your vagus nerve for self-regulation, then, you are able to develop the capacity to activate your vagus nerve at will. You will be able to encourage your body to trigger that parasympathetic reaction at will. Your body will naturally calm. Your heart rate and blood pressure will regulate. Your body will begin to rest. This will lead to more restful sleep, allowing you to better digest the food that you do ingest. You will be able to make sure you are at your best, all because of the vagus nerve.

Despite the fact that this nerve is relatively unknown to the general public that has not had a reason to look into it, whether because they are thankfully healthy or they simply have never heard of it before, it is incredibly important to understand. If you have ever felt like you struggle with your physical or mental health, it is entirely possible that learning about your vagus nerve, learning to activate it, could enable you to overcome those feelings of malaise. You can learn to alleviate your suffering, encouraging yourself to relax far more than you ever thought was possible. This is fantastic—it means that you can care for yourself. You can relax. You can take your health and wellbeing into your own hands, and when it is in your own hands, you are more likely to feel like it is meaningful. Having control of that, learning to activate your vagus nerve for health and relaxation purposes can then enable you to live the best life you can.

As you continue to read this book, you will be introduced to several exercises that will activate your vagus nerve. In activating the vagus nerve, you will then be able to trigger all of the benefits that have briefly been discussed, though you will see a more in-depth understanding of the myriad of ways activating your vagus nerve can and will help you in the future. With the techniques provided in Part III, you should be able to activate your vagus nerve on your own.

Chapter 3: History of the Vagus Nerve

For the longest time, people were unsure how the body regulated itself. It was unknown how the body was capable of an awareness that would disappear after death, or how the brain processed and communicated with the body. People did not know how the nerves and muscles communicated, only positing that they did. However, with time, a man's dream, and some dissecting of frogs, it was discovered that largely, nerves communicate through neurotransmitters.

The Discovery of Neurotransmitters and the Vagus Nerve

After a dream in 1921, Otto Loewi dissected two hearts out of two frogs—one kept the vagus nerve while the other did not. The hearts were kept beating and were bathed in saline solution. The heart with the nerve attached was then stimulated, naturally causing the slowing of the heart rate as the vagus nerve activated. That liquid was then suctioned from the first heart with the slower heart rate and bathed onto the other, which had no vagus nerve attached. It slowed as well in response to the saline solution that had first been exposed to the stimulation of the vagus nerve.

The neurotransmitters, in particular, acetylcholine, allowed for the nerves to communicate, triggering the nerves to send down the powerful impulse down the line and to the next nerve, through which more neurotransmitters would be released. These neurotransmitters became readily available in the saline solution and then triggered the same expected responses in the heart without the vagus nerve, all because the neurotransmitters were still present without it. This allowed Loewi to come to the understanding that it was not through electrical impulses that nerves communicated with muscles, though electrical impulses were still important to nerves themselves—they communicated with the muscles through the creation and secretion of chemicals.

This was the beginning of understanding how nerves worked—it was obvious that the impulses of the nerves were both electrical and chemical. This is crucial in the later development of the vagus nerve stimulators that are known to the world today, allowing for the literal electrical stimulation of the nerves present. Before delving further, however, we need to stop and consider what vagus nerve stimulation typically consists of when not triggered by an individual and instead is created through medical devices.

Vagus Nerve Stimulation Devices

With the understanding of how powerful the vagus nerve is, recognizing just how crucial it is to regulate the human body, experiments have been done regarding whether the vagus nerve could simply be stimulated on demand, allowing for the creation of the effect necessary. After all, if it is the neurotransmitter acetylcholine that creates the triggering the parasympathetic nervous system, and you can trigger the creation of that neurotransmitter as simply as applying a shock to the vagus nerve, as Loewi demonstrated when studying the hearts of frogs, it should be possible to create that same effect in humans.

Thus, the concept of the vagus nerve stimulator was created.

Originally designed to be used as an alternative plan for the treatment of seizures, particularly in epilepsy patients, treatment of humans with vagus nerve stimulation became reality in 1988. However, it was studied in animals far earlier—back in the 1950s, it was found to prevent seizure activity in cats with feline epilepsy, and then later found effective in canine epilepsy as well. Throughout the years and species, it was found that triggering the vagus nerve did, in fact, treat the seizure.

In the 1980s, then, humans began being implanted with the vagus nerve stimulator, a small device that is implanted into the body and attached to the vagus nerve. It works through triggering the electrical impulse necessary to activate the vagus nerve. Because the vagus nerve is afferent, meaning it returns signals to the brain, the vagus nerve stimulator essentially provides shocks to the nerve, which acts as a sort of pacemaker to the brain. They lessen the severity of epilepsy, though they do not actually cure epilepsy. Generally speaking, people find that they are incredibly beneficial.

Vagus Nerve Stimulation at Home

Over time, it became more understood just how integral the vagus nerve is—it plays a part in several key areas of the brain and body, and because of that, it has become an area of interest for those interested in holistic medicine, treating the whole body rather than just whatever organ is problematic at that moment in time. The vagus nerve, when it is out of sorts and not regulating itself well, can cause a wide array of issues. It can lead to increased anxiety, depression, PTSD, arthritis, and more, all because the vagus nerve regulates so much of the body. Without the stimulation necessary, or without the toning of the vagal pathways that are necessary, you can find that your entire body suffers. You may find that you cannot sleep, or that your digestion is all out of sorts.

Instead of looking and treating those specific symptoms, such as prescribing a sleeping aid or encouraging an elimination diet, it is entirely possible that what is needed is for those involved to stop and consider whether they need to instead treat the whole body. Is it possible that symptoms of insomnia or indigestion are coming from another part of the body?

It absolutely is.

The brain is in control of the entire body. It regulates everything from your breathing to your temperature. It controls your digestive processes, whether you are digesting food in the first place, and even functions such as the liver or intestines. Everything originates in the brain, and without the brain, those functions will not work. Of course, the signals that go between the body and brain are directly related to the vagus nerve, one of the cerebral nerves. It then stands to reason that potentially, the problem may not simply be insomnia or indigestion, but rather that the messages between the body and brain are being mixed up and misread at some point. There may be a miscommunication there somewhere that is causing the problems.

Of course, when there is a disconnect between the body and mind, it is time to start considering which nerve system may be responsible for that. When considering the different pathologies that will be discussed within this book, the root is typically the vagus nerve. The vagus nerve is responsible for connecting the body's function back to the brain, communicating what is happening or supposed to be happening. If the vagus nerve is overactive or underactive, it will not be effective. Messages will be distorted in some way, and there will become some need for a change somewhere along the way.

This is where vagus nerve stimulation comes in. People have found that there are several ways to trigger vagus nerve stimulation, and these can be used in order to ensure that the individual that is suffering can get the most relief possible. As you continue to read, you will be introduced to the problems that a faulty, overly active, or underactive vagus nerve can cause. Part II is dedicated entirely to looking over these pathologies, relating them back to the vagus nerve and creating that solid foundation and understanding of them. This, then, enables the individual to understand that what they may need is to jump-start that nerve, triggering it themselves.

Chapter 4: The Vagus Nerve and the Nervous System

As a nerve, you would be entirely correct to identify the vagus nerve as a part of the nervous system. After all, it is literally in the name. Despite how complex the human nervous system is, understanding the basics will not only benefit you on this journey of understanding how and why you should activate your vagus nerve, but also how it is actually working within you. Understanding the drastic effects of a few simple gestures and actions can really help drive the point home—activating your vagus nerve can really impact your entire body.

Components of the Nervous System

At the simplest, your nervous system comprises of several different pieces that work together to create the nervous system. The most fundamental are the neurons, ganglia the brain, and the spine. These communicate largely through neurotransmitters and action potential. Now, this section is only going to give you a brief overview of what each of these parts does, rather than going into extreme depth. If you are interested in learning to develop a deeper understanding of these concepts, you may benefit from looking at biopsychology in depth.

However, considering this is a book primarily about the vagus nerve, you will get just enough information to understand the function of these four key players in the nervous system.

Neurons

These are the most fundamental units within the nervous system. Think of these as individual building blocks of the nervous system as a whole. Every cell within both the central and peripheral nervous system are comprised of neurons. These are what communicate throughout the body—they transfer information to and from the brain, allowing for the functioning of the human body as a whole. When you are discussing neurons, there are three major types: Motor neurons, sensory neurons, and interneurons.

Your motor neurons are largely responsible for communication to parts of the body that need to function. You will see communication from the brain telling different body parts how to work. They allow for the functioning of glands, muscles, and organs the way that they should be.

Your sensory neurons are responsible for anything you sense. Your sensory organs—the nose, eyes, mouth, ears, and skin, are able to sense what is going on around you, and that information is sent to the brain through the peripheral nervous system, first traveling to the spine and then to the brain, where it is then processed.

Your interneurons are the sort of intermediaries—they go between motor and sensory neurons, allowing for communication of what to do next. For example, if you touch something that is hot, your sensory neurons are able to communicate to your motor neurons that you need to move through the interneurons.

Motor Neurons
- Communication between body parts-- glands, muscles, organs, etc.

Sensory Neurons
- Communication from sensory organs to the spinal colum and brain

Interneurons
- Intermediary between sensory and motor neurons

The Brain

The brain behaves as the processor—it is where all information comes in, gets processed, and then it sends out information for the body to proceed accordingly. Effectively, the brain tells the body what to do next with information that the body sends to it. It is recognized to have three major areas: the forebrain that is capable of processing any sensory information, problem solving, and conscious thought, the midbrain that is associated with the processing of hearing, sound, and movement, and the hindbrain that processes unconscious actions like breathing, heart rate, and balance.

Of course, there are other areas to the brain as well—it can be broken into several much smaller anatomical parts, but again, for the purpose of this book, you do not need to go into too much depth with the biology of the brain.

The Spinal Cord

Another major portion of the nervous system is composed of the spinal cord. This is a long series of nerves that go from the brainstem all the way down the length of the spinal column. The spinal cord, along with the brain, creates the central nervous system. It is responsible for communicating nerve impulses to and from the brain. Afferent nerve pulses from the extremities are able to go to the brain at this point, while the brain is also able to send impulses through the spine to those extremities.

The Ganglia

A ganglion (plural: Ganglia) is a cluster of nerve cells. Typically, these are outside of the central nervous system, instead of being found primarily in the autonomic nervous system. They can be both sensory and autonomic and serve as a sort of relay for information. Sensory ganglia send information to the brain from the peripheral nervous system whereas autonomic ganglia send information from the brain to the body.

Neurotransmitters

Neurotransmitters are the chemicals that are released after an electrical impulse has gone down the length of a neuron. These neurotransmitters allow for the activation of the next neuron in line, allowing for the communication across neurons and throughout the body. When the neurotransmitters are received, they trigger an action potential, allowing for the cycle to continue.

Action potential

The action potential is the discharge of an electrochemical in response to the neurotransmitters that were received by the previous neuron in the path. These are either triggered or they are not—there is no middle ground or partial triggering of a neuron into an action potential discharge. The action potential is the electrical response to the chemical neurotransmitters. When you read about an impulse, you are reading about an action potential, or activation of that particular nerve.

Central Nervous System

The central nervous system (CNS) refers primarily to the brain and spine—this is the part of the body that is responsible for gathering, processing, and responding to outside stimuli. Nerves gather information throughout the peripheral nervous system, centralize that information to the spine and brain, and the brain can then process it.

This is the part of the body that is going to make up the bulk of the nervous system—it senses what is happening around you and responds to it, as well as what keeps you alive. You need your CNS to survive and function. Damage to this can cause damage to your ability to function. Severing the spinal cord at certain areas can lead to paralysis, or even death, and brain damage can cause extensive personality and ability shifts or death. Damaging a certain area of the brain can mean sudden death, while damaging others could eliminate an individual's ability to speak coherently, see, or even breathe, depending on which part of the brain becomes damaged in the first place.

Peripheral Nervous System

The peripheral nervous system, despite the fact that it is not the brain, is a bit more involved than much of what you have seen thus far. The peripheral nervous system (PNS) is everything that is not the spine and brainstem—it is all of the nerves that are interlaced throughout your body. Your vagus nerve falls into this category because, despite the fact that it originates in the brain, the vagus nerve also extends beyond either the brain or the spine, venturing through the body and down to the abdomen.

The peripheral nervous system can be divided up further. Take a look at this table to see just how the peripheral nervous system can be divided:

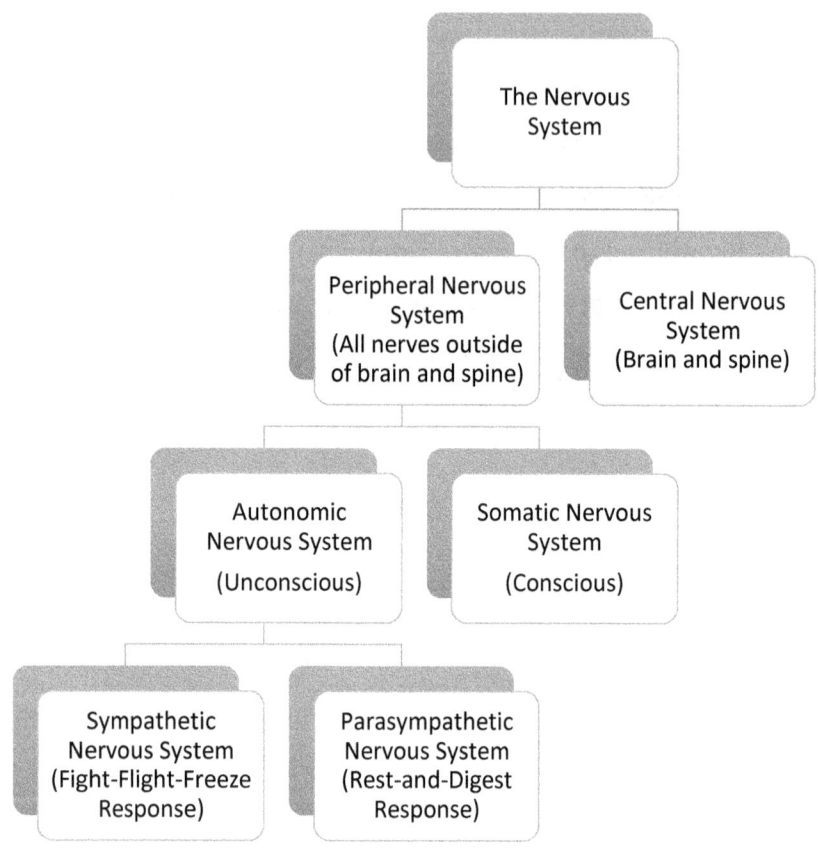

Autonomic vs. somatic nervous system

Your PNS is first divided into either autonomic or somatic functions. The autonomic functions are largely unconscious—they are entirely involuntary. These may be the production of information between internal organs and the brain, such as regulating the heart to beat and the lungs to breathe.

On the other hand, the somatic nervous system is voluntary—these are impulses related to sensory input. This is the sensation you get through your skin and your ability to move your muscles in order to control your body. While you cannot control your heartbeat at will, you can control where your body goes and what it does—you can choose to walk, run, jump, or dance, for example. While your choice in actions can influence your heart and breathing rate, they will not control it.

Your vagus nerve falls into the autonomic nervous system—it is directly related to the control of systems that are unconscious and involuntary.

Sympathetic vs parasympathetic nervous system

The autonomic system can be broken down even further. As you know, the autonomic system is already unconscious. It has two modes that it uses to regulate how it will run the organs: these are controlled by the sympathetic and parasympathetic nervous systems. When the body is stressed or threatened, the sympathetic nervous system takes over. This is your fight-flight-freeze response, in which you respond strongly and viscerally to the possibility of being threatened and attempt to do anything you can to survive. You may choose to run away from a threat that you feel you cannot defeat. You may choose to fight off a threat you feel like you can contend with. You may even completely freeze if your mind is entirely overwhelmed by the threat—your mind shuts down, saving you from the suffering of what it assumes will be a death. This is what triggers deer or rabbits to suddenly freeze up when they are terrified—it is their minds' way of protecting them.

The parasympathetic nervous system, on the other hand, rules the body during times of relaxation. This is your rest and digest state—this is where you are able to get proper rest in and ensure that you are actually digesting your food effectively. When the sympathetic nervous system is in control of the body, your system is so concerned with surviving that moment rather than surviving long term that you are not getting the proper rest or the proper digestion. This can lead to serious long-term issues—you can run into anxiety, depression, insomnia, PTSD, and more, all because your body gets caught into a loop of being stuck in the sympathetic nervous system.

Of course, as discussed already, your vagus nerve controls the parasympathetic nervous system. The activation of your vagus nerve should be able to switch the body over to the parasympathetic nervous system, creating the state of rest-and-digest instead of fight-flight-freeze.

Chapter 5: The Vagus Nerve and the Body

As with all of the nervous system, the vagus system works in tandem with the body—it can influence the body in ways that are shocking. Despite being a single pair of nerves, the vagus nerve system is capable on influencing several parts of the body, thanks to its role in influencing and controlling the autonomic nervous system. It is directly related to the heart, lungs, and digestive system, and because of that, it is able to have a massive impact on the body and physical symptoms that one may feel. While this chapter will not be discussing issues related to these parts of the body, it will touch upon the influence of the vagus nerve and stimulation of the vagus nerve with these parts and functions of the body.

Location of the Vagus Nerve

Within the body, the vagus nerve leaves the brain and goes down the neck, traveling between the carotid artery and jugular vein down into the abdomen. From there, it reaches outwards throughout the body. It branches outward to other nerves in the peripheral nervous system, and eventually reaches down as far as the colon. Between 80 and 90% of the body's afferent nerves return to the vagus nerve, which then communicates with the brain.

As it goes down the body, the vagus nerve travels down the neck, passing by both the esophagus and trachea before reaching the heart, at which point it branches out to the heart, lungs, and the esophageal plexus. It continues down, entering the diaphragm and the abdomen, at which point it is able to interact with the digestive system.

As you can see, it absolutely warrants the name of wanderer considering just how far it travels throughout the body and just how much of the peripheral nervous system it consists of. The vagus nerve, then, becomes incredibly important due to its overarching reach across the body and the fact that it consists of nearly all of the afferent nerves that return back to the brain, communicating with it. This means that the vagus nerve, if it does not function perfectly, is going to cause struggles simply because of the fact that so much of the brain's information is routed through it. It is connected to several of the most essential parts of the body that are crucial to your survival, and because of that, it becomes one of the most important nerves within your body.

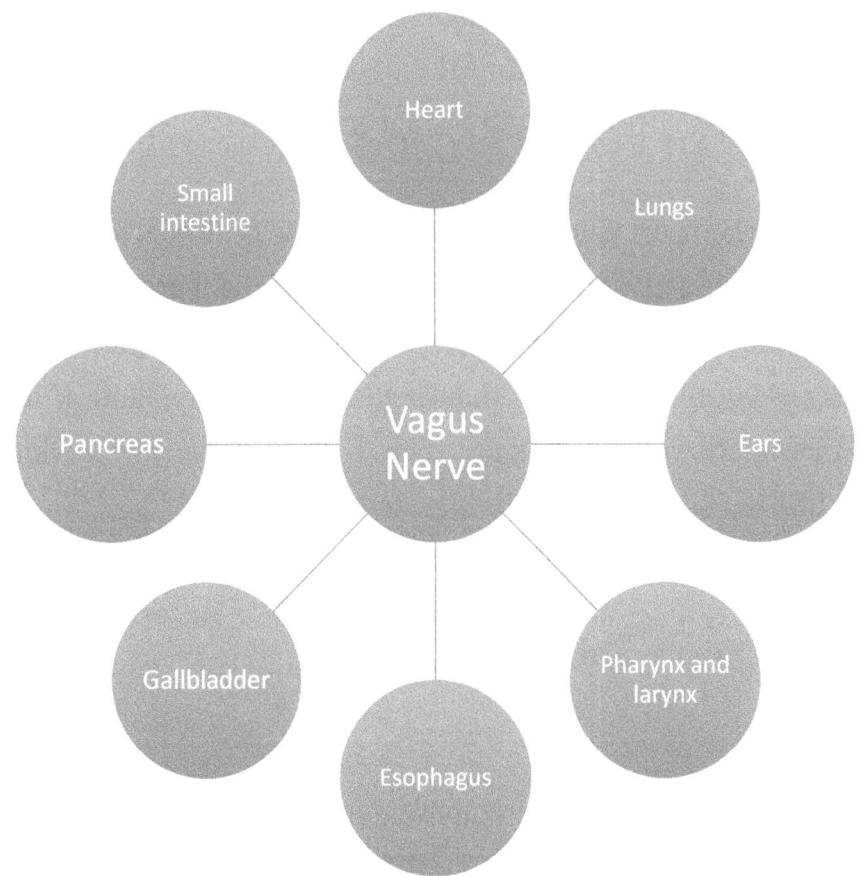

Vagus Nerve and the Heart

The vagus nerve is entirely capable of regulating the heart rate. The stimulation of the vagus nerve then triggers certain muscles within the heart that cause the heart rate, and therefore blood pressure, to drop. Your vagus nerve directly impacts the production of acetylcholine, which is what is involved in regulating the heart rate. It slows the pulse. Of course, on the other end of the spectrum, if the vagus nerve is not stimulated enough, the heart rate would be higher.

Because the heart rate is a major predictor of how stressed the body is, the activation in relation to fight-flight-freeze should come as no surprise. The body, when activating the sympathetic nervous system, triggers that higher heart rate, and if the parasympathetic system is not there to reduce the rate at which the heart is beating, it will be elevated.

Vagus Nerve and the Lungs

Similarly to the heart, the vagus nerve is directly related to respiration. As it is so closely related to the heart and heart rate, it should be no surprise that it is similarly intertwined with the breathing rate. In fact, the same acetylcholine that is used to slow the heart is important to the breathing process. It also connects to the diaphragm, allowing for further influence over breathing rates.

In particular, the vagus nerve, when active, tells the brain to constrict bronchi present in the lungs. This, of course, means that breathing becomes more difficult. However, deep breathing, on the other hand, can trigger the vagus nerve to report that the body is calm, leading to a state of relaxation. This, then, means that the lungs are one way to trigger the vagus nerve without relying on electricity.

Vagus Nerve and the Digestive System

As a major component of the parasympathetic nervous system, it should be no surprise that the vagus nerve is intimately linked to the digestive system as well. Remember, the parasympathetic nervous system is linked to the rest-and-digest mode—when it is active and regulating the organs, it encourages the digestion of food. When your vagus nerve has your body in parasympathetic mode instead of allowing the sympathetic nervous system control, your body is able to digest food with less issue—it will directly communicate with the stomach and intestines that food should be pushed through.

Essentially, the vagus nerve controls the muscles within the digestive system that are responsible for contracting to push and process food within it. When the vagus nerve is functioning normally, this is no problem—food will travel at a normal rate and be digested as it normally would. However, when the vagus nerve is not working for some reason, whether it has become damaged or is simply not functioning at that moment due to being caught in fight-flight-freeze mode, food remains in the stomach.

Of course, this does not have very good end results—the food that lingers can very possibly rot and become a breeding ground for all sorts of bacteria that can cause issues.

Vagus Nerve and the Inflammatory Reflex

The vagus nerve is directly responsible for the inflammatory reflex. This means that it is responsible for the regulation of whether the body needs to create an immune response to fight off an infection of some sort of whether it needs to create inflammation. When there is some sort of injury or infection, this information gets passed to the brain, which in turn triggers the vagus nerve. The vagus nerve then communicates with the spleen, encouraging it to release the immune system. It tells the body to regulate the inflammatory reflex when it functions normally.

However, when the vagus nerve is not functioning properly, the inflammation can go awry—it can carry on far more than is healthy or acceptable, leading to inflammation in the body. It can also reduce itself too much, leading to an immune system that struggles to cope with any sort of heavy load on it. This means, then, that the body cannot manage any sort of illness and may frequently become ill as a result.

The Vagus Nerve and the Body

As it becomes apparent, the vagus nerve is essential when it is functioning properly. The body is able to self-regulate, running like the well-oiled machine that evolution has created. On the other hand, if it is overactive or underactive, you can start to run into problems. It can drastically influence the body in several ways, all because it was so crucial in the first place. At the end of the day, you want to ensure that your vagus nerve is functioning properly. This can happen for any reason—sometimes for no reason at all. Nevertheless, through reading this book, you will be able to start identifying patterns that can be useful for you to understand, and you will learn several ways that you can start regulating your vagus nerve once and for all.

Chapter 6: The Vagus Nerve and the Mind

Along with its myriad of effects on the body, the vagus nerve can also cause some serious impacts on the mind as well. As you read through this chapter, you will see several ways that the vagus nerve directly and indirectly can influence the mind. Of course, the vagus nerve is part of the unconscious portion of the nervous system, but it is still surprisingly active in several processes that have a direct impact on your conscious processes and state of mind.

Most people do not think of the ways that their bodies may directly influence their minds, but in reality, it does plenty. You go through a cycle of thoughts creating feelings, which create behaviors, which then directly influence your thoughts more. This sort of cycle is never-ending—meaning you can directly influence your mind through your body. That is what your vagus nerve does; it takes the cues from your body and transfers them to your mind. Whether you become aware of those thoughts or not may be a different story, but your behaviors can directly influence them.

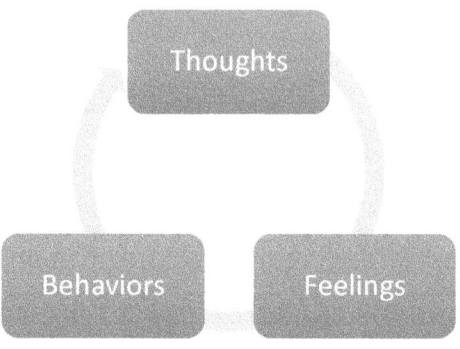

The Vagus Nerve and Memories

The vagus nerve has been found to influence the creation of memories—linking the production of norepinephrine. As the vagus nerve is responsible for regulating the sympathetic and parasympathetic nervous systems, when it has triggered the sympathetic system to function, it causes a release of norepinephrine. This seems to show that small levels of stress can actually be beneficial to the body in terms of making memories.

In a study done by the University of Virginia on rats, it was found that stimulating the vagus nerve triggered the release of norepinephrine into the amygdala. This is a portion of the brain largely related to memory storage. The stress, then, triggered the rats to lock onto those memories, finding them to be consolidated. Essentially, the vagus nerve recognizes when the body produces epinephrine, a neurotransmitter that is released in the fight-flight-freeze response within the body, then triggering the release of norepinephrine within the brain.

The Vagus Nerve and Relaxation

On the other hand, the vagus nerve can also trigger the release of acetylcholine in order to trigger the shift from the sympathetic nervous system to the parasympathetic nervous system. Of course, the acetylcholine has already been discussed and confirmed to be directly related to the creation of a slower heart rate and deeper breathing, both of which can trigger a sensation of relaxation.

Beyond acetylcholine however, the vagus nerve is also able to trigger the release of other neurotransmitters, such as oxytocin, vasopressin, and prolactin, all of which can aid in relaxation and reward cycles, mostly related to the reproductive cycle. Oxytocin is a reward neurotransmitter most commonly associated with orgasm, though it is also related to bonding after having a child among other acts. Oxytocin is the pair-bonding hormone in humans, encouraging a deeper and more meaningful relationship. Vasopressin regulates the sexual motivation felt, something that can only be triggered when you are in rest-and-digest mode, which is sometimes also called feed-and-breed. Prolactin is triggered by pregnant and breastfeeding women, allowing for the production of milk. When women are stressed, they cannot produce prolactin—in fact stressful stimuli or events can actually trigger a woman to start drying up instead of continuing to produce milk.

The Vagus Nerve and Gut Reactions

Everyone has gut reactions sometimes—you know what they are. That feeling when you feel like you know something is wrong in the pit of your stomach. This is because the gut and the mind are closely linked—in fact, the microbiome within your gut is believed to be closely related to your mind. This is believed to be due to the vagus nerve—it sends signals from the bacteria to the brain.

Effectively, your vagus nerve is responsible for the gut reactions you feel. The next time you realize you are feeling uncomfortable walking down the alley and try to brush off that pit of dread in your stomach, realize that you are trying to silence one of the most influential nerves in your body, and that it is entirely possible that the gut is having that feeling for a very good reason and you should listen to it.

The Vagus Nerve and Fight-Flight-Freeze

Thanks to its role in the autonomic nervous system, the vagus nerve is closely linked to fight-flight-freeze responses, in which you are inundated with fear and stress and suddenly have a strong impulse to either fight your way into survival, run for your life, or freeze entirely, hoping that the attacker will lose interest or assume that you are already dead in the first place. This, of course, directly impacts your mental state—it can trigger intense feelings of fear, which may then become anger if you start moving toward fight mode.

This means, then, that the vagus nerve can have some impact on your emotional state, particularly relating to feeling negative motivating feelings, such as fear and anger.

The Vagus Nerve and Rest-and-Digest

On the other hand, your vagus nerve can trigger the parasympathetic response instead, urging your body to put the brakes on that gross overreaction and instead trigger your body to relax. This triggers your body to enter what is known as rest-and-digest mode. During this state, your body is no longer frantically attempting to funnel your energy and blood into your extremities, preparing to keep yourself alive. This then means that your body will be more relaxed in general. You will feel better-rested, and better-nourished, as you will come to find that even your digestive system slows and regulates itself out.

This, of course, then leaves you in a much better mental state than you were before. You will be able to relax, feeling like you are safe and comfortable because you no longer have your sympathetic nervous system screaming at you to jump into action as soon as possible. You are no longer guided by the anxiety and fear that your sympathetic nervous system triggers and instead can focus on whatever you actually legitimately enjoy instead.

Neurotransmitters and the Vagus Nerve

At this point, there have been several neurotransmitters discussed throughout this book. Let's take a quick recap of the ones that have been discussed. Think of this chart as a quick guide to the neurotransmitters that have been relevant thus far. Keep in mind that these are simplified explanations of each neurotransmitter, and they do not consider the fact that there are several other functions possible with these neurotransmitters—this is focusing entirely on the relationship of these neurotransmitters with the vagus nerve.

Acetylcholine
- Controls the contraction of muscles. Is related to the vagus nerve and triggers a slowing of the heart rate

Epinephrine
- A stress hormone also known as adrenaline-- increases heart rate and glucose in blood

Norepinephrine
- Stress hormone in the brain-- it triggers alertnes, memory consolidation, and anxiety

Oxytocin
- Reward hormone involved in bonding in relationships, sexual behavior, and bonding with children after childbirth

Prolactin
- Relevant to women who are activley breastfeeding children or are pregnant- it creates the bonding between mother and child

Vasopressin
- Regulates bodily functions, used in response to pain, and relevant to sexual function, particularly in men

Part II
Pathologies of the Vagus Nerve

Chapter 7: The Vagus Nerve and Anxiety

Have you ever had that feeling that something is not right? You may not be able to put a finger on it, but you have that feeling of imminent dread, as if something is lurking just around the corner and no matter how certain you are that there is nothing there or that you are being irrational, you cannot help but feel worried. No amount of telling your mind that you are overreacting is enough—you still feel like there is some sort of threat lurking around the corner.

If that sounds familiar, it is entirely possible that you could be suffering from anxiety. This means that your body is constantly feeling as though there is some imminent threat lurking around the corner, no matter how irrational it may be.

What is Anxiety?

Anxiety itself is one of the most common mental health issues in the world. While anxiety on its own is sometimes normal, healthy, and totally expected, such as if you are going to your first day at a new job, or if you have a job interview, it is important to understand that if your anxiety has become such a constant in your life that you are always struggling, always suffering, and always attempting to get out from underneath that stress, it could be a problem in your life.

When you are anxious, your fear drive is on auto-pilot. You may feel a sense of dread deep within yourself that you cannot explain or regulate. You may feel like you have no way to stop those feelings of fear and dread, and oftentimes, it can be incredibly difficult to do so if you are not armed and prepared. Sometimes, it could be a dull pang, a quiet whisper in the back of your mind telling you that you are not good enough, but other times, it can be so extreme, so detrimental, that you find yourself legitimately panicking for no reason. It can manifest as phobias, as obsessions and compulsions, or as panic attacks. Other times, it can manifest as just a deep-seated feeling of dread and terror. Nevertheless, it is important to recognize just how that anxiety can impact your life.

Anxiety Disorders

Anxiety comes in several different forms, as already briefly mentioned. These disorders can be more or less invasive in your life, depending on the severity of the symptoms you are feeling or having. Nevertheless, they all are related to some sort of sense of anxiety, leading to feelings of a loss of control, like your life is in danger or being threatened, and directly influencing your ability to function effectively within your life. You may struggle with day-to-day tasks simply because of the severity of your symptoms.

Before we move on to symptoms, let's take a look at some of the most common forms of anxiety disorders:

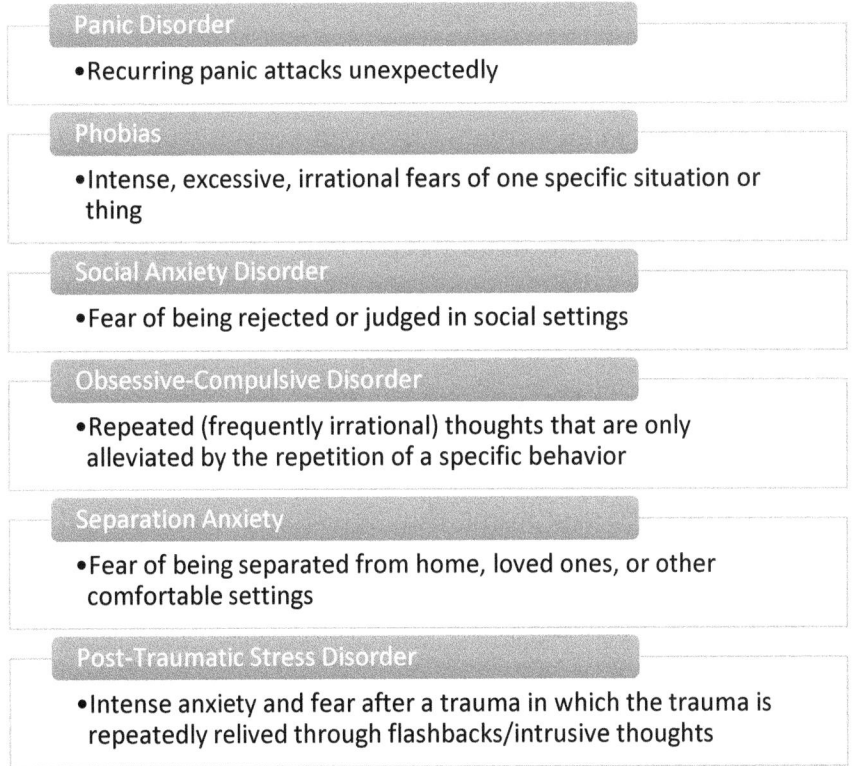

While this is not an exhaustive list of anxiety disorders, it does cover the general idea of the most commonly suffered disorders. Again, please keep in mind that the disclosure of these disorders and lists of symptoms does not substitute seeing a properly licensed medical professional if you feel like you may legitimately be suffering from an anxiety disorder. If you feel like you may have anxiety disorders of any kind, please make an appointment with your primary care provider.

Anxiety Symptoms

Anxiety symptoms can vary greatly from person to person. Each person will feel anxiety in a different way from those around them. This means that some people will report having several different symptoms of anxiety, while others will report having none. There are no specific symptoms or presentation of symptoms that must be present in order to diagnose—in order to get a diagnosis, rather, you must show that you have any number of anxiety symptoms that are severe enough that they are directly impacting your life for the worse. These symptoms can include the following:

- **Sweating, with or without chills and/or hot flashes:** Sometimes you can feel like you are suddenly sweating or freezing, even though you were perfectly comfortable moments ago

- **Shakiness or trembling:** Often shakiness goes hand-in-hand with anxiety, even if you have no reason to feel anxious at that moment

- **Feeling as if you are choking or short of breath:** Especially during anxiety or panic attacks, you may suddenly feel like you are choking or struggling to breathe

- **Chest pain, with or without heart palpitations:** Oftentimes, people with anxiety will struggle with heart palpitations—this is the feeling of a racing heart. It may or may not come along with chest pain as well

- **Dizziness, with or without tingling throughout the body:** Especially during an anxiety attack, the body may suddenly feel like it is tingling or numb, like a pins and needles sensation while you, yourself, feel dizzy

- **Detaching from the world around you:** Especially during an anxiety attack, you can feel like you are no longer in touch with the world. You may feel like you are drifting, or like you are not actually you, as if you are living in a dream

- **Nausea:** Anxiety can frequently bring about nausea

- **Fear of death or imminent danger:** When you are anxious, you can feel like you are facing imminent demise or like you are going to die or be hurt in the very near future

- **Difficulty concentrating:** When you are anxious, it can be hard to focus your mind on what you are trying to do or what you need to get done

- **Emotional regulation issues:** When struggling with your anxiety, you can struggle to keep your mood in check. You can go from just fine one moment to suddenly furious for no real reason at the drop of a hat

- **Changes in sleep:** When you suffer from anxiety, you can struggle with your sleep. Sometimes, you may sleep too much, while others, you may struggle with insomnia and not being able to sleep at all

- **Changes in personality:** Sometimes, people find that their personality starts to shift, especially when the anxiety leads to strongly avoiding certain hobbies or events. The anxiety can also become overwhelming and make the individual listless and fearful

- **Fatigue and restlessness:** Despite the constant insomnia and desiring to sleep, the individual may find him or herself constantly feeling restless and unable to get comfortable to sleep in the first place

- **Avoidance of areas or stimuli:** Particularly for those with phobias or PTSD, people can find themselves avoiding areas that they believe will trigger particularly strong emotions or flashbacks

- **Hypervigilance:** The constant state of anxiety can lead to feeling like you constantly have to look over your shoulder or be on edge in case something comes out to hurt you

Anxiety and the Vagus Nerve

As already well-established, the vagus nerve activates the parasympathetic nervous system to create the rest-and-digest state for your body. A lack of the vagus nerve activating, then, allows for the sympathetic nervous system to run amok, allowed to rule the body altogether. It creates an increase in stress hormones, which then triggers inflammation, which can impact the brain.

Beyond that, however, the longer the sympathetic nervous system is allowed to rule, the more stressed and anxious the body becomes, creating higher levels of cortisol and glutamate, both of which stress out the body even further. This means that you are left feeling miserable.

The vagus nerve, of course, is going to be sending impulses back to your brain to fill it in with how the body is feeling, due to its afferent status. The longer this stress goes on as well, the less likely it is that the parasympathetic nervous system will kick into play in the first place, meaning that you will be less likely to be able to defeat that anxiety at any given point in time. Unless you are able to kick-start your vagus nerve back in gear to get it moving, you are going to struggle.

Chapter 8: The Vagus Nerve and Depression

Along with anxiety, another commonly occurring mental health issue is depression. When you feel depressed, you may struggle with your own thoughts. Many people around the world struggle with depression, with an estimated 300 million people suffering. It is nearly as common as anxiety, and of those people, nearly 50% of them also get diagnosed with an anxiety disorder as well, leading to a double hit of mental health issues all at one time, causing serious struggle for them. At any given point, roughly 15% of the adult population will go through some sort of depressive episode during their life. It is incredibly common—if you think that you may be suffering from depression, know that you are not alone.

What is Depression?

Depression is characterized by the negative feelings associated with it. Those suffering from depression at any point in time feel as though they are sad or hopeless much of the time. They may struggle to find interest, value, or purpose in most things that they are doing at any given point in time, and because of that, they struggle to function. As they grow more and more depressed, they struggle further and further with interacting with other people. They cannot manage the life that they once did, feeling as though their ability to focus has gone away, and even if they could focus, they would find little use in doing so in the first place.

Depression itself comes in many different shapes and forms, ranging from major depressive episodes to seasonal affective disorder. Each of these can have their own impacts on one's life, however, and even mild depression is just as worthy of treatment as major depressive disorders.

In order to be diagnosed with depression, the symptoms of depression must be persistent and consistent, lasting at least 2 weeks in which symptoms are severe. Those with more mild depression are oftentimes likely to take much longer for diagnosis than those who have severe depressive disorder.

Despite the fact that depression seems to hit women twice as often as men, possibly due to hormone fluctuations related to the menstrual cycle and pregnancies of women, anyone can suffer from depression. Adult or child, man or women, anyone can potentially suffer, and when they are left without treatment, it could last for months or years.

Depression Disorders

Depression disorders come in many different forms. While all of these will vary I severity and symptoms, they all cause very real distress and discomfort to the individual suffering from the feelings in the first place. Because of that, it is important to go through with speaking to a doctor if you suspect that you may have depression. Nevertheless, here is a list of the most common depressive disorders:

Seasonal Affective Disorder
- These people see depressive symptoms associated with the change in seasons. Most common in northern areas in which sunlight is scarce in the winter

Postpartum Depression
- Depression that is triggered after the birth of a baby

Major Depressive Disorder
- A severe form of depression in which the individual suffers from intense feelings of sadness

Dysthymia
- Mild, persistent depression that may last for years

Depression Symptoms

Depression, despite the myriad of symptoms that it brings about with it, is largely treatable. You can get relief from these symptoms, whether through medication, learning to regulate your vagus nerve in hopes of alleviating symptoms, learning to manage through therapy, or any other treatment method that is discussed between you and a doctor. Please remember—if you ever feel as though you are thinking about harming yourself, you should treat this as a medical emergency and you should seek out emergency treatment immediately.

- **Low mood:** When you are depressed, you almost always struggle to function effectively. Your mood fails to regulate and you feel down the vast majority of the time. Keep in mind that those are depressed may not always show signs of depression 100% of the time—they may be depressed some of the time but seem fine the rest of the time. It is entirely dependent on the individual that is being considered at that moment in time.
- **Change in appetite:** You may find yourself endlessly hungry or entirely uninterested in eating altogether thanks to your depression.
- **Sleep disturbances:** As with eating, you may find yourself sleeping constantly or not at all. You may find

yourself suffering from extreme insomnia or feeling the urge to sleep constantly without ever feeling rested.
- **Irritated and agitated:** You fail to regulate your mood regularly due to the fact that you are constantly depressed and feeling negative. Those negative feelings very quickly give way to irritation when things do not go your way.
- **Fatigued:** No matter how much sleep you may get, you always feel exhausted and fatigued. Sometimes, even getting out of bed can seem like too much effort.
- **Struggling to concentrate:** You frequently struggle to concentrate, feeling like your mind is sluggish and struggling to function.
- **Lack of interest:** Everything that used to bring you enjoyment and pleasure now seems bland and dull in comparison. You find little to no pleasure in anything that you could possibly do.
- **Feelings of guilt and worthlessness:** You may feel as though you are worthless or guilty of something that you did not do in the first place, despite the fact that you do not have anything to feel guilty for. Especially if you are struggling to function on a daily basis, you may feel like you are letting your friends and family down.
- **Fixation on death or suicide:** You may self-harm, or you may strongly consider suicide, and may even spend time coming up with plans to make those thoughts a reality, even if that is not something you feel like you

would ever go through with. Sometimes, the hopelessness can just seem too overwhelming.

Depression and the Vagus Nerve

Despite the fact that most forms of depression can be treated with less invasive methods, the fact that vagus nerve stimulation can treat depression implies that there is some involvement there. While it is not entirely known why stimulating the vagus nerve will trigger an improvement in depression, especially treatment resistant depression that has been difficult to treat in the first place, it has been found to be effective.

This should come as little to no surprise—the vagus nerve is responsible for managing the relaxed state in which people are able to rest. However, just as with anxiety, when the vagus nerve is unable to trigger the parasympathetic nervous system to rule the body, the sympathetic nervous system is allowed to reign supreme over the body, wreaking its havoc as it continues for too long. Just as with anything, moderation is key—some stress is good, and can even be motivational, but when the sympathetic nervous system is free to rule the mind, inflammation begins to occur.

That inflammation in particular could potentially be related to depression. It has been found that those with this increase in inflammation can lead to the depressed mood. The inflammation lessens serotonin levels within the brain, which then leads to mood regulation problems. After all, depression is commonly treated with selective serotonin reuptake inhibiters (SSRIs), which create larger concentrations of serotonin in the brain to combat the symptoms altogether.

The implication, then, is that the lack of stimulation from the vagus nerve allows the sympathetic nervous system to run rampant. That causes an inflammatory response within the body, which then also creates the response in which the body struggles to produce enough serotonin. That lack of serotonin, then, is linked to the depressive symptoms.

Chapter 9: The Vagus Nerve and Chronic Illness

Chronic illnesses are problematic for those who suffer from them—they involve long-term suffering, and can create significant issues for those who are suffering. When suffering from chronic illnesses, people run into several issues, ranging from struggling to cope with medical bills as a result of treating their conditions in the first place to attempting just to get by in life while actively suffering. These chronic illnesses can impact all sorts of areas in life, influencing whether someone is able to get through their day to day tasks in some way.

It has been shown that as much as six in every ten adults currently living within the United States of America are suffering from a chronic disease of some sort—that is 60% of adults within the country. Perhaps even more staggering twenty-five in one hundred have at least two, but oftentimes more chronic illnesses. Stop and think about your close friends and family for a moment—60% of them likely suffer from at least one chronic disease, and 25% likely suffer from more than one. This means that the majority of people that you will meet are suffering one way or another.

What are Chronic Illnesses?

Chronic illnesses are relatively vague—there are several entirely unrelated diseases and conditions that could be considered chronic. In order to be considered chronic, there are a few criteria that must be met: the condition must be long-lasting, require medical care, and/or it may limit daily activities and functioning.

- Long-lasting (at least one year)
- Require medical attention
- Can limit daily functioning

These illnesses and diseases, despite the fact that they are long-lasting and limiting, are still not always fatal. Chronic illnesses are largely considered to be manageable, and while they absolutely do directly impact your quality of life, they do not necessarily condemn you to an early death. You can live an entire, mostly whole, life with a chronic illness that is being effectively managed by a medical professional with a treatment plan that works for you.

Effectively, chronic illnesses are usually considered to be illnesses or conditions that are long-lasting. Despite the fact that they sometimes come with remission stages, in which the sufferer remains relatively symptom free, people usually see a relapse after which the symptoms return. These illnesses can be contagious or entirely non-communicable, depending on the condition in particular.

Often, when you see "chronic condition" used to describe something, it is usually describing some sort of syndrome, any sort of impairment, a disability, or a disease. So long as it meets the criteria, it will be considered a chronic condition.

Common Chronic Illnesses

Chronic illnesses and conditions, like the people who suffer from them, come in a wide variety of shapes and sizes. These can include anything from cancer to HIV, with nearly everything in between considered a chronic ailment. Some of these can be problems with pain while others can mental health issues. Others still can lead to a degradation of the body's ability to function effectively. Overall, the type of the chronic illness can range greatly. In fact, all of the conditions that you will be reading about within this book can be considered chronic.

Nevertheless, let's take a brief look over three common chronic illnesses that people suffer from. As you go through these illnesses, try to identify the ways that they may be related to the vagus nerve.

Alzheimer's disease

Alzheimer's disease is a form of dementia—when someone suffers from Alzheimer's, they often start out with mild memory loss that eventually progresses to debilitating levels. Usually, it appears after age 60, but it is possible for younger people to suffer from the disease as well. It is not considered normal, nor to be expected through aging. What it does, however, is disrupt daily life and can require the individual suffering from it to require long-term or around-the-clock care by licensed medical professionals.

While it is not entirely known what causes Alzheimer's, it is believed that a common link between age, genetics, and physical health are related to the development. There is currently evidence that high blood pressure and cholesterol may be responsible for raising the chances for ever developing the disease, and that certain activities, such as socializing, exercising the brain, and physically exercising yourself can lessen the risk.

It cannot be cured, but it can be managed in the hopes of providing the individual with the best life possible for the duration of their years. The use of vagus nerve stimulation is being researched as a possible treatment for Alzheimer's disease, showing that there are changes in quality of life for those who are treated with the stimulation.

Obesity

Though it is not commonly considered a disease, obesity is more than a superficial occurrence—it is not just about looks, but about health as well. When you are obese, you risk developing a myriad of other health issues, ranging from heart disease to cancer. Those who suffer from obesity have excess body fat, and for some people, that weight is harder to shed than for others.

With obesity, your body mass index (BMI) is rated at or above 30—25-29.9 is considered overweight, 18.5-24.9 is considered normal, and anything under 18.5 is considered underweight. Of course, the BMI is not perfect—it does not account for variants in skeletal size or muscle density.

Obesity has all sorts of risk factors—it could be caused due to hormones, genetics, or simply bad habits, such as eating too much without exercising. Oftentimes, those who are obese eat more than those who are of healthy sizes, and may also eat due to their own feelings as a way to sort of self-soothe.

Diabetes

Diabetes itself refers to several disease that all alter how your body processes glucose—the primary substance used for energy by your body. Typically, when considering diabetes, you will be looking at two disease: Type 1 diabetes and type 2 diabetes. These two diseases vary greatly. Women can also develop gestational diabetes as a result of a pregnancy.

Type 1 Diabetes

- The pancreas produces little or no insulin, which the body uses to allow cells to utilize glucose. This is genetic and often manifests in childhood.

Type 2 Diabetes

- The body starts to resist insulin or struggles to produce enough insulin. This is largely impacted by lifestyle-- being overweight and sedentary can directly influence your likelihood of developing this disease.

Gestational Diabetes

- This form of diabetes develops during prengancy-- the hormones produced by the placenta cause a resistance to insulin, which can lead to blood sugar levels lingering too high for pregnancy. This is usually develped at the end of pregnancy and goes away after birth.

These diseases can wreak havoc on the human body, directly influencing how the body functions, heals, and regulates itself. Considering that we primarily eat to raise blood sugar in order to continue functioning at a normal level, having that disconnect and struggle for the body to regulate accordingly can lead to massive issues. The body sometimes struggles to function and heal, and if left untreated without care taken to treat the diseases, it can lead to neuropathy and eventually death. Blood sugar levels that rise too much can cause comas and even death.

The Vagus Nerve and Chronic Illness

The vagus nerve relates to all three of these illnesses—if you stop and look at some of the symptoms, you can start to piece this together on your own. Alzheimer's disease sufferers start to see legitimate progress with their cognitive abilities and anxiety related symptoms when they have their vagal nerve stimulated. While it is not entirely known why, it is known that several of the precursor risk factors to Alzheimer's are related to the vagus nerve—high blood pressure can make it more likely that it is developed later in life, which as you know, is linked to the vagus nerve.

When it comes to obesity, the vagus nerve regulates the digestive system. This means that the individual's digestive system is going to respond to the vagus nerve. It will entirely regulate based on feedback by the vagus nerve—the nerve will determine whether your brain receives the message that you have eaten your fill or not, which then impacts how much you eat. Obesity, ultimately, is usually associated with the vagus nerve losing sensitivity for some reason—having a poorly responding vagus nerve means that the signal that tells your brain that you are full is too quiet. Effectively, then, the vagus nerve's dysfunction can, in some instances, be attributed to the obesity.

Diabetes, then, can also be closely linked to the vagus nerve—if it regulates the diet, and some diabetes can be induced via diet, it stands to reason that diabetes is sometimes caused by the vagus nerve. Beyond just that, however, the vagus nerve, at least in mice, has been found to provide information to the brain about the glucose levels within the body. Therefore, if that informational circuit were to get damaged, it would become vastly more difficult to regulate whether the individual had a sufficient level of glucose in the blood.

Chapter 10: The Vagus Nerve and Inflammation

Inflammation is not inherently a bad thing—it is a defense mechanism that the body employs to protect and heal the body. It is, essentially, a sign that your body is fighting off some sort of foreign body. This may be bacteria, or it could be a virus, or even something that has fallen out of place. Despite being a normal response by the immune system, it can also cause a myriad of issues as well, if allowed to get out of hand. It can cause pain, stiffness, and even struggles to function if the immune system goes overboard.

What is Inflammation?

As simply put as possible, inflammation is swelling in the body. The area swells and warms and the body then knows to focus on healing that particular area. It could be some sort of injury or an infection from bacteria—no matter what it is, inflammation is how the body triggers itself to go and pay attention to the area in order to ensure it heals. Without this inflammation, the body would not heal in a timely manner—your broken bone would never mend itself and your infections would be free to run rampant like an invasive species, destroying the area around them and quickly spreading to infect more of you.

Effectively, if your body is a vehicle for your mind, think of your inflammation as your maintenance system. It will go through, flag areas of concern, and then work on healing it. Of course, it can also be overzealous as well. As with all things in life, there is such thing as too much of a good thing—when left to its own devises and free to worsen as much as it wants, inflammation can cause massive issues. It can lead to all sorts of autoimmune diseases and disorders, in which the body begins to attack itself instead of only on harmful injuries and foreign bodies.

Step 1: Infection or Injury
- At this stage, bacteria or a foreign object has infected the body

Step 2: Activation of Macrophages
- The body sends out macrophages to start fighting against bacteria as a first defense before white blood cells arrive on the scene

Step 3: Dilation of Blood Vessels
- The conflict between the immune systems and the bacteria create chemicals that dilate the blood vessels. This allows more blood to arrive, allowingfor more white blood vessels to fight off the infection-- this is where the signs of inflammation appear

Step 4: Dendritic Cells Arrive
- This communicates to the body which cells need to be activated in order to handle the infection-- they differentiate between a need to fight a virus or bacterial infection

Step 5: The Army Arrives
- At this point, with the information from dendritic cells, the proper attacking force arrives to fight off the infection

Step 6: Recovery
- At this point, your body starts to heal. White blood cells remove themselves, allowing for swelling to go down.

Effectively, as you can see dictated in the previously provided table with a step-by-step play of the inflammation cycle, it is meant to directly protect and heal the body from any infections. In fighting off the bacteria and viruses that are causing problems, the body is providing itself with a chance to repair damage before it festers and gets out of hand. This means that the individual is able to recover from infections that, if left ignored and untreated, could be fatal.

Symptoms of Inflammation

This inflammation, however, is not without side effects or symptoms. Especially when inflammation goes from acute, or temporary, to chronic, it becomes more and more of a strain on the human body. Usually, this chronic inflammation is caused by the body thinking that there is a problem or a threat to its wellbeing somewhere, despite the noted absence of any such points. Nevertheless, whether your inflammation is chronic or acute, you will find similar symptoms, such as:

- **Mild fever, with or without chills:** Fever allows the immune system to continue working by making the body less hospitable to any perceived threats

- **Feeling tired or fatigued:** Because the body is using more energy to attack any problematic areas, there is less energy available for you. This leads to sleep, which also promotes further healing at a quicker rate

- **Stiffness, particularly around the area of inflammation:** Any joints that are actively being attacked by inflammation will sometimes stiffen—as more and more swelling presents itself, moving the joint becomes difficult

- **Joint pain or swollen joints, which may be warm:** Similarly, the swelling and inflammation can lead to the joints hurting and feeling warm to the touch—these are telltale signs that the particular joint is being attacked by the immune system, either to treat an already present injury or because an injury is perceived

- **Loss of appetite:** Due to the cytokines, the substance secreted by the cells of the immune system, and how they interact with the brain, the individual who is suffering from inflammation usually sees a decrease in appetite

- **Struggling to use or move the impacted joint:** Similarly to the stiffness found in the joint, the individual may struggle to actually use the joint during an inflammation attack—it becomes difficult or even impossible to fully use the join in some instances until the inflammation goes away

Inflammation Disorders

Inflammation is largely associated with arthritis in particular—while not all forms of arthritis are associated with misfiring immune systems, three particular forms of arthritis are: Rheumatoid arthritis, psoriatic arthritis, and gouty arthritis are all forms of arthritis that are directly related to inflammation. There are other disorders that are directly related to inflammation as well, and there are also other forms of arthritis that are not necessarily associated with inflammation, so keep that in mind.

The three forms of arthritis that do relate to inflammation, however, can be incredibly painful. While rheumatoid arthritis in particular will get a chapter to itself (Chapter 16), it is important to understand all three of these forms of arthritis caused by inflammation gone awry.

Psoriatic arthritis is specific to people who are already suffering from psoriasis—which is a type of skin condition that results in skin that appears red, patchy, and with greyish-silver scales developing atop them. Those who suffer from psoriasis sometimes also develop psoriatic arthritis, in which your immune system attacks itself. It most often results in the swelling of fingers and toes, feeling pain within your feet, particularly where connective tissue meets bone, and pain in the lower back. This particular kind of arthritis can do serious damage to the joints, largely because the immune system is effectively targeting the joint that is healthy—despite the absence of a threat or danger, the area is attacked due to the inflammation.

Gouty arthritis, sometimes just known as gout, is a type of arthritis that is the result of uric acid levels being too high.

Essentially, the uric acid solidifies within the joints, and the solid crystals of uric acid tend to form into sharp points, which then can hurt the joint. As the joint becomes hurt, then, it develops the common symptoms of arthritis as a result.

Inflammation and the Vagus Nerve

Since the vagus nerve is the primary source for the body and brain to communicate, allowing for feedback in both directions, it is primarily responsible for identifying when there is inflammation within the body. When it is able to find that inflammation, largely through detecting cytokines, the brain finds out about that inflammation and can then make sure that the proper amount of anti-inflammatory hormones are released. This means that the inflammation is properly regulated—it is not too strong, nor is it to underwhelming.

This proper response leads to people with entirely normal, functioning inflammation levels when it is necessary. For example, when you are injured or you get a minor infection, that inflammation is necessary. The body regulates itself. However, for some people, this inflammation response can be largely suppressed, leading to immunodeficiency. Those whose response is too strong, on the other hand, can find themselves struggling with highly responsive inflammatory responses that attack themselves.

Chapter 11: The Vagus Nerve and PTSD

People tend to associate PTSD solely with war veterans, but you do not have to be in a soldier to suffer from this form of anxiety—anyone who has endured some sort of trauma, either experiencing or happening to witness whatever has happened, can suffer from PTSD. As a direct result of that trauma, the individual may find that he or she is struggling with their trauma. While it is normal for people to feel upset with what has happened to them and struggle at first, most people tend to bounce back. However, for other people, the feelings of hopelessness, terror, and overall inability to cope never improve, or even get worse in some situations. Those people are told that they may have PTSD, which rarely goes away on its own.

What is PTSD?

Short for post-traumatic stress disorder, PTSD is a form of anxiety. Usually triggered by some sort of horror, it typically involves a massive struggle to cope with some sort of trauma, whether that trauma was intentionally inflicted or entirely coincidental. People can suffer from PTSD after a car accident, losing someone close to them unexpectedly, losing a home, particularly when unexpected and violent, being the victim of some sort of assault, physical or sexual, enduring abuse, or really anything else that would potentially be traumatic for the individual.

Those who struggle with PTSD often find themselves facing flashbacks and recurring intrusive thoughts that can make coping effectively nearly impossible. They essentially get stuck in a cycle in which the brain cannot properly process and handle the traumas, and as a result, they find that they are unable to finally get themselves out of fight-flight-freeze mode and back into rest-and-digest mode. Because of this, those suffering from PTSD can seem especially volatile, especially in situations or contexts that are even vaguely reminiscent of the trauma they endured. In fact, even something as simple as a scent, a word, or the way something is said can trigger an attack if the individual is reminded of the trauma in some way.

It is important to note that those who suffer from PTSD sometimes have feelings that they are better off hurting themselves or even ending their lives. These suicidal thoughts, tendencies, and ideations should be taken incredibly seriously and as a medical emergency. If you feel like you are having suicidal thoughts or feelings, it is important that you reach out to someone you can trust—perhaps a friend, family member, or spouse, and ask for help. You do not have to feel this way forever, and there is no reason to create a permanent solution to something that is temporary at worst. If you have no one you can reach out to, please do not hesitate to call your emergency services for help.

Symptoms of PTSD

The symptoms of PTSD can primarily be broken down into four distinct categories: These are intrusive memories, avoidance, negative changes to one's thought processes and general affect, and changes to how one physically and emotionally reacts, sometimes known as arousal symptoms. Each of these categories can present in different ways and all of them can cause hugely negative implications if allowed to fester and worsen without intervention.

Intrusive thoughts can encompass several different symptoms on its own, all summed up into that one little phrase. Those who are suffering from intrusive thoughts find themselves struggling to control their own thoughts. For some, they may dwell on the past while others find themselves lost in flashbacks of the trauma, feeling like they are stuck reliving it. They may have nightmares, and oftentimes, they will directly respond with largely irrational reactions when something similar or reminiscent to the trauma is encountered.

Avoidance largely encompasses the act of making it a point to entirely avoid anything that even remotely relates to the trauma. For some, this is actively refusing to speak about what has happened, carrying on like nothing ever happened while still avoiding what has happened. Some people will even make it a point to change schedules, routines, and anything else necessary to entirely avoid the situation at hand. They will do everything possible to accommodate their feelings, even though doing so is largely unhealthy and completely subverts healing at all.

Mood changes also occur regularly with PTSD—the individual suffering from the condition may find him or herself feeling as though they are worthless or at fault for some reason. Moods fall and they start feeling largely negative about themselves and the world. As their affect changes, their relationships may start to struggle as well—they will feel detached from their loved ones, and because of that, they also struggle to maintain their relationships. Memory problems can also crop up, especially relating to the trauma in particular, and they can find themselves feeling numb much of the time, or struggling to feel positive emotions at all.

Lastly, people suffering from PTSD tend to struggle with physical reactions as well—they may find that their startle reflex is on overdrive and they are constantly on guard, even when situations do not call for it. They may engage in behaviors that are considered reckless, such as drinking heavily or driving too quickly, and they may struggle to get enough sleep and concentrate. They may also struggle with emotional changes as well, such as finding themselves far more aggravated than usual, or feeling intense guilt.

PTSD tends to vary over time—it can be incredibly tense at first, or suddenly seem to almost go away, only for the individual to find that they are suffering with the thoughts once more. The individual may be entirely fine one moment, only to fall apart at the sound of something happening around you. If you find that you are having recurring intrusive thoughts or flashbacks that are making functioning difficult for you, it is important that you should see your doctor, especially if these thoughts have lasted longer than a month after the trauma you have endured. With diagnosis, you can put together an action plan to protect and care for yourself.

Post-Traumatic Stress Disorder Symptoms

Intrusive Thoughts:	Avoidance:	Negative Changes to Mood:	Arousal Symptoms:
•Flashbacks and unwanted memories of the trauma that are unavoidable •Nightmares about the trauma •Reacting strongly and emotionally to anything reminiscent of the trauma	•Actively attempting to avoid thoughts or topics of conversation related to the trauma •Actively avoiding anywhere related to the trauma •Changing schedules to accommodate the trauma	•Low self-worth •Struggling with memory •Struggling with relationships with friends and family •Losing interest n things that once brought joy •Struggling with positive emotions	•Heightened startle reflex •Being guarded •Struggling to sleep •Feeling angry, aggressive, ashamed, or guilty •Engaging in self-destructive behaviors

PTSD and the Vagus Nerve

Keep in mind just how intricately linked to fight-flight-freeze and rest-and-digest the vagus nerve is and consider for a moment what PTSD is. It involves regulating the fear response, as well as telling the body when that fear response is appropriate. If PTSD is largely due to an inability to regulate those responses to the trauma, it stands to reason that the two are intricately linked to each other.

Evidence has shown that those suffering from PTSD do, in fact, show a diminished functioning of the parasympathetic nervous system, implying that it is not regulating itself effectively and because the body is never able to put the individual into rest-and-digest mode due to the lack of the parasympathetic activity triggering the proper hormones, instead the individual is stuck in fight-flight-freeze mode. Consider the symptoms for a moment: Feeling guarded and afraid are two major symptoms of PTSD, and both of them are directly related to the sympathetic nervous system being in control. Now consider insomnia, which is an inability to sleep. That inability to sleep is related to the fact that the body cannot get itself out of fight-flight-freeze mode. During that time, the individual is stuck awake, no matter how tired he or she may be feeling, all because the body is unable to relax enough to effectively sleep.

When the parasympathetic nervous system takes control defensively, as is common in PTSD, the body shuts down on itself. It overcorrects, leading to a numbness or freeze response. Then, with people with PTSD, they are reacting with an overactive or underactive vagus nerve, leading to that feeling of shutting down and being numb or unable to feel joy.

Chapter 12: The Vagus Nerve and Autoimmune Disease

Autoimmune disease and the vagus nerve are just as closely linked as inflammation and the vagus nerve. A part of this is because inflammation and autoimmune issues are intricately related—inflammation is an autoimmune response. A handful of autoimmune issues have already been discussed thus far—you have learned about arthritis and diabetes. However, there are several other autoimmune diseases that people can suffer from as well.

Immune disorders can go either way—it can result from an overactive immune system or an immune system that is not active enough. Either way, there are issues with the body managing its own illnesses as the defense systems fail one way or the other. The end result is that some part of the body fails to engage in fighting off the illness, infection, or other trigger for the body.

The Immune System

The immune system is the system through which the body can defend itself from illness or infection. It consists of several different types of white blood cells. There are phagocytes, which attack the bacteria or virus that have infiltrated the body. Lymphocytes, another variety of white blood cells, then document the structure of the virus or bacteria, allowing the body to remember the problematic invader and prevent it from arising in the future. Both phagocytes and lymphocytes can come in various forms, with each and every one acting as a specialized soldier for the job—some are trained to do generic care while other are more specialized. For example B lymphocytes lock onto targets that need to be defeated before signaling that the system needs help.

The immune system works in several ways—it creates three different forms of immunity. People can have what is known as innate immunity, adaptive immunity, or passive immunity. Each of these function differently, but the result is the body having a defense against some form of disease. Depending on which it is, people that have each form have a slightly different form of immunity with slightly different impact.

Innate Immunity

- This is what people are born with-- it is the skin, which acts as a primary fortification against any sort of illness or disease. From there, the base immune system itself, with its ability to recognize foreign bodies, is an innate immunity.

Adaptive Immunity

- This is what people develop over time-- for example, when you get a vaccine, you build an adaptive immunity. As your body fights off different illnesses, it produces necessary defenss, which function as an adaptive immunity.

Passive Immunity

- This is immunity that is built up temporarily. For example, when a baby drinks breast milk, he or she absorbs antibodies, which the provide the baby with antibodies necessary to stay safe.

What is Autoimmune Disease?

Autoimmune diseases are forms of disease that develop when the immune system does not function properly, and instead, becomes overactive. During periods of being overactive and running rampant, the immune system attacks the body instead of anything toxic or dangerous. This then directly damages the body, causing injury, inflammation, and suffering.

This means, then, that the best way to treat an autoimmune disease is to find a way to slow down and reduce the immune system, and in doing so, the flare-up of the autoimmune disease should fade away, allowing for relief. Some of these autoimmune diseases will only cause problems in one area of the body, while others can impact everything, creating feelings of discomfort and suffering. Nevertheless, regardless of the harm that whichever autoimmune issue you are suffering from causes, it becomes important to treat to ensure that the body is preserved in the best possible condition for you.

Some of these tendencies for creating autoimmune issues can be directly related to genetics with studies linking them to the families, while it is believed that diet and exercise can also cause autoimmune disorders. One last thought process on why these diseases are developed is called the hygiene hypothesis—this hypothesis posits that due to the fact that children are exposed to far less germs now than they ever were before, due to immunizations becoming commonplace and the development of sanitizing cleaners that kill off the germs that children would have otherwise impacted, the immune system develops a tendency to overreact. Effectively, because the immune system is not being triggered on the regular, it becomes faulty. Despite this theory, however, it is currently unknown what for sure makes people prone to disorders or why they develop they do.

Common Autoimmune Issues

Of the autoimmune issues that you could suffer from, there are over 80. Some of these are more common while others are practically unknown. Of those 80, 14 are relatively common. These disorders are common enough, for the most part, that you can mention them and people will have at the very least heard of them. These 14 diseases include:

- **Rheumatoid Arthritis:** A disease in which the immune system targets joints, causing stiffness, pain, and inflammation in the joints that have been targeted.
- **Celiac Disease:** A disease in which the immune system directly attacks the digestive system, leading to gastrointestinal sensitivity and inflammation.
- **Sjögren's Syndrome:** A disease in which the immune system attacks the glands within the eyes that create the tears and lubrication. It is most commonly seen as dry eyes and mouth.
- **Addison's Disease:** A disease in which the adrenal glands are unable to produce the proper rates of hormones, leading to the body beginning to malfunction.
- **Hashimoto's Thyroiditis:** A disease in which the thyroid does not produce enough hormones. It then leads

to weight gain, struggling to tolerate the cold, goiter, and losing hair.

- **Psoriatic Arthritis:** A disease in which the immune system causes the skin to develop too quickly—the excess skin develops in patches that become inflamed and scaly. Arthritis sometimes goes along with that psoriasis, leading to joint pains and problems.
- **Pernicious Anemia:** A disease in which the body does not get enough protein and struggles to produce DNA effectively.
- **Inflammatory Bowel Disease:** A disease commonly referred to as IBD in which the immune system targets the intestinal wall. This can present in several different forms that lead to inflammation of the GI tract, leading to pain and difficulty digesting food properly.
- **Autoimmune Vasculitis:** A disease in which the immune system impacts the blood vessels in the body, leading to inflammation of the vessels, which then causes the veins and arteries to become more narrow, simultaneously making the blood flow more difficult as well.
- **Multiple Sclerosis:** A disease in which the immune system targets the brain—particularly the myelin sheath, which is the part of neurons that coats the axon to bolster transmission of the impulse. As this becomes damaged,

the individual's effectiveness at passing along messages becomes decreased.

- **Graves' Disease:** A disease in which the immune system attacks the thyroid, leading to too many hormones being produced and released into the body. This can lead to high heart rates, struggling to tolerate heat, and unexplained weight loss.
- **Myasthenia Gravis:** A disease in which the immune system damages the way that the brain communicates with the muscles by impacting the nerves that communicate from mind to body, leading to muscle weakening that seems to be worse when more action is gone through.
- **Systemic Lupus Erythematosus:** A disease in which the immune system attacks much of the body, targeting the brain, joints, several organs, and even the heart. It leads to rashes, pain, and fatigue.
- **Type 1 Diabetes:** A disease in which the immune system targets cells within the pancreas that are responsible for the production of insulin, causing the body to no longer process glucose effectively.

Autoimmune Disease and the Vagus Nerve

Remember, as discussed, the vagus nerve directly informs the brain when there is inflammation somewhere in the body so the body can then influence just how much inflammation is allowed. However, when the vagus nerve becomes damaged, it is not capable of protecting the body from the inflammation. This means the inflammation is free to run rampant, creating all sorts of havoc for the body, all because the vagus nerve malfunctioned in some way.

Stop for a moment and consider all of the implications that this can have, and recognize the sheer number of people that find that they are suffering from an autoimmune disease—upwards of 8% of population are believed to suffer from an autoimmune disorder. 8 people of every 100 that you pass are likely suffering from their autoimmune disorders malfunctioning in some way, and because of that, their body is directly attacking themselves.

Stimulation of the vagus nerve, however, has been shown to help fight inflammation, which then should also help alleviate some of the autoimmune response. With the inflammation limited, the body is no longer sending cues to tackle parts of the body that did not require an actual intervention from the immune system in the first place.

Effectively, the afferent path, the path from the body to the brain, communicates to the body whether there is currently an injury or a need for the inflammation and immune response in the first place. It has been found that when the afferent nerve is blocked in some way, but the efferent pathway is free to continue as normal, or even stimulated, the body is able to regulate itself. It allows for the continued communication from the brain to the body while stopping the brain from producing more hormones that encourage inflammation because it is not receiving the impulses that are telling the brain that inflammation is happening and needs to continue in the first place. In blocking the afferent while encouraging the efferent impulses, the body has a chance to regulate itself—it stops producing the cytokines that are going to create further inflammation that is responsible for the attack of the body by the immune system.

Chapter 13: The Vagus Nerve and Fibromyalgia

Fibromyalgia is quite painful for those who suffer from it—it is currently far more likely to be diagnosed in women than men, and those who have fibromyalgia are also more likely to have several other disorders than those who do not. Despite how much is currently known about fibromyalgia, the cause itself is not yet understood. What is understood, however, is that it creates the sensation of pain, likely due to it amplifying the pain response. Sensations that would ordinarily be tolerable can feel painful to the individual with fibromyalgia, and the pain that is felt can then cause several other issues as well.

What is Fibromyalgia?

Despite what people may frequently believe, fibromyalgia is not an autoimmune disorder. It is a condition that is linked to feeling pain, and despite the similarities to many autoimmune disorders, it is not yet believed to be caused by the immune system attacking itself. The evidence to prove the production of autoantibodies, the antibodies that have developed the tendency to attack their own body, or seeing any harm that can be caused by the suffering of fibromyalgia, it does not quite fit the necessary qualifications to be defined as an autoimmune disorder in the first place. However, several autoimmune disorders can be experienced while simultaneously suffering from fibromyalgia—they are occur regularly enough in tandem that it is being studied. Nevertheless, fibromyalgia itself is not seen to have a direct impact on the physical body.

Despite this fact, however, fibromyalgia is a very real condition. While it is not seen physically and is not particularly easy to diagnose or observe, there is no denying that the pain is real. It can be seen to run in families, which implies that it may be genetic. There have also been links between specific illnesses and infections and the development of fibromyalgia. It has even been found to suddenly arise after some sort of physiological trauma, and even stress can trigger it to occur.

Symptoms of Fibromyalgia

There are three key symptoms of fibromyalgia that arise and are present to allow for a diagnosis. These three symptoms are pain, fatigue, and struggling cognitively, at least some of the time. Aside from those three symptoms, however, it has been found to be linked to several other conditions and disorders as well, including but not limited to IBS, migraines, and TMJ disorders.

The pain associated with fibromyalgia is largely widespread—it is felt constantly and throughout the body. In order to warrant that diagnosis of widespread, it must happen on both the left and right sides of the body, and above and below the waistline. When it is felt in all four quadrants of the body, it can be considered to be widespread. This must be constant or near constant for at least three months, and those who suffer from it describe it as a dull ache that never goes away.

The fatigue associated with fibromyalgia is reported, regardless of how much is slept. It is quite possible that, due to the pain, the individuals do not sleep well, and therefore are not getting the rest that they need in order to really feel like they have gotten enough. Because of the pain, they may have other sleep disorders. It is not uncommon to see those with fibromyalgia also reporting that they have restless leg syndrome or sleep apnea as well.

The cognitive difficulties that the individuals with fibromyalgia describe get commonly referred to as "fibro fog." This is the feeling that the individual cannot focus on what they are supposed to, and it can be debilitating. Focusing on work, necessary tasks, or even just getting through chores can be incredibly difficult, all because those suffering from the condition cannot muster up the mental power to remain focused.

It is not yet known why it is that people with fibromyalgia hurt, but it is believed that something happens that changes how the nerves are functioning. Through repeated stimulation of specific nerves in the brain, it is believed that neurotransmitters increase to reach an abnormal level, and when that happens, the pain then is felt more frequently. As this pain is felt, the individual then begins to become more sensitive to the pain as well, as if it is essentially habituated and primed to react in this manner, and the pain receptors then end up more sensitive than intended, linking to the sensation and overreaction of the brain to trigger pain responses.

Fibromyalgia and the Vagus Nerve

As with many of the other conditions which have been discussed thus far, it has been seen that the triggering of the vagus nerve stimulates the parasympathetic nervous system, which then directly reduces the sympathetic nervous system. Due to the fact that the vagus nerve can lessen the fight-flight-freeze response, it is able to effectively push the hormones necessary to reduce those stress hormones, allowing for an alleviation of symptoms.

In those suffering from fibromyalgia, it has been discovered that the parasympathetic system is not functioning as well as it should be. This can be studied by looking at the heart rate variability—the amount by which the heart rate fluctuates during breathing. Heart rates, despite what people tend to believe, are meant to be irregular. Try looking at this for a moment—find your pulse. When you take in a deep breath, you should notice that your heart rate quickens as you inhale. As you exhale, you should notice that your heart rate slows.

Effectively, you want a higher heart rate variable (HRV) to show that your entire autonomic nervous system is functioning effectively. The sympathetic and parasympathetic nervous systems are functioning together, and when your HRV is higher, you show that you have a toned vagal nerve, meaning it is functioning properly.

The parasympathetic nervous system regulates your heart rate—without it, your heart rate would linger somewhere around 100 bpm on its own. Instead, however, the vagus nerve regulates that out, which also causes variations in the heartbeat, and because the parasympathetic nervous system can really only regulate a handful of beats at any given moment, the heart rate comes out as inconsistent. The sympathetic nervous system, on the other hand, increases the heart rate, and because the heart rate is increased, there is far less time that any sort of irregularity could occur, and this lasts much longer than the parasympathetic influence. Essentially, then, the most healthy autonomic nervous systems are those with a lower heart rate and a higher HRV, showing that the parasympathetic nervous system is regulating the heart rate.

Due to those suffering from fibromyalgia showing reduced activity in their parasympathetic nervous system, then, it becomes clear that there is an increase in sympathetic nervous system's control over the individual's body. This, then, implies that the pain may be related to that dysfunction of the parasympathetic nervous system, which is a dysfunction of the vagus nerve itself.

Chapter 14: The Vagus Nerve and Sleep Disorders

Sleep: When you were a child, you hated it, and as an adult, you probably wish you had more of it. Your body needs it to function, and a massive portion of your life will be spent slept away. You will effectively spend about 33 YEARS of your life in a bed either trying to fall asleep or actually sleeping. Think about how long your life span really is—roughly 79 years in the United States, and you are spending almost ½ of that either in a bed or actively sleeping.

Of course, some people struggle to sleep effectively—they may have insomnia or simply have bad sleep hygiene. Nevertheless, the effects of sleep deprivation are incredibly real and noticeable after a relatively short period of time. It takes only about 20 hours before the body starts to show noticeable signs of sleep deprivation. Before we continue on with this chapter, however, let's stop and take a look at what sleep actually is in the first place.

Sleep

Despite common perceptions, sleep is not just a time for the brain to turn off for the night—it actually facilitates several different processes that are necessary for proper functioning. Sleep is largely found to have three key functions: It allows the body to recover, it facilitates the memory consolidation process, and is related to the immune system. Each of these three functions are crucial, and are so important that the human body happens to spend about 1/3 of each and every day actively asleep, not counting the time preparing to sleep and getting comfortable in order to all asleep. Sleep is important, and if you do not give it to yourself, your body will eventually force the point—you will fall asleep at some point, even if you try to stay awake in the first place.

When you sleep, your body repairs itself. Your cells are literally attempting to regenerate themselves, and the rest of your body slows down so energy can be redirected to those cells that need it, allowing them to heal themselves. As you sleep as well, your mind begins to consolidate all of the memories you have made throughout the day, also allowing you to effectively learn better. It has been found that those who sleep shortly after being taught to play a video game tend to do better than those who stay up late in an attempt to practice longer to develop skills quicker.

Lastly, when you sleep while sick, your body is able to better produce cytokines, allowing the body to then fight off the infection quicker, which is quite likely why people get so tired when they are sick.

Sleep		
Facilitates restoration of the body	Allows for better learning and memory consolidation	Enables better immune response when sick

What are Sleep Disorders?

Sleep disorders, then, are the creation of some change in the way that you are sleeping, and these changes are typically quite negative. They can involve sleeping too much, not enough, or simply not getting restful sleep in the first place. The end result to not getting enough sleep, however, is the creation of all sorts of health issues. Sleep deprivation itself can quite literally be dangerous, especially because the signs of sleep deprivation can be so extreme.

Some of these symptoms include mood irregularities, creating irritation and depression. They can lead to cognitive impairments, causing a struggle to concentrate on any tasks at hand and forgetfulness, as well as a struggle to learn anything new, and more. The effects are more than just physical—they are mental, as well, and those mental impairments can be deadly if you were to, for example, try to drive while severely sleep deprived. Studies that have been performed have shown that driving after having been awake for at least 17 hours is equivalent to driving with a blood alcohol level of 0.05%, which is just under the 0.08% that is sited as cause for drunk driving.

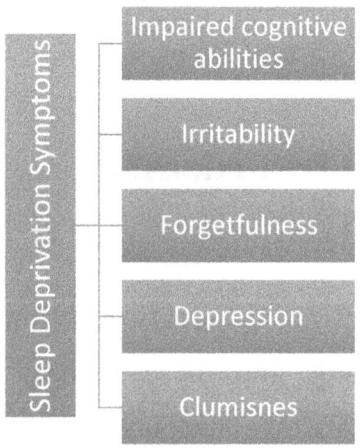

Of course, the implication of this is that sleep disorders, which are constantly stripping away at your sleep will cause a myriad of issues for you—you will find your performance and ability to function impaired, all because of your lack of sleep. Sleep disorders can vary from person to person and type to type, but within the vast majority of these sleep disorders, you are not getting enough sleep.

Common Sleep Disorders

Sleep disorders vary from type to type, but there are several that exist. This particular section will look at sleep disorders that are believed to be related, at least in some way, to the vagus nerve. These all share similar symptoms—you will likely be sleepy during the day and may struggle to fall asleep or stay asleep at night. Some people will also go on to fall asleep during times that are considered dangerous or inappropriate, such as at work or even when driving a car.

- **Insomnia:** When you suffer from insomnia, you usually either struggle to sleep at night or you cannot stay asleep at night. You may find yourself regularly waking up, despite your best efforts to clean up your sleep hygiene.

- **Sleep apnea:** When you suffer from sleep apnea, your breathing patterns when asleep are abnormal. This can be due to some sort of neurological issue, or also because you have slept in a strange position or are obese and have an obstruction of your windpipe when in lying down positions. This is something that most people do not notice when they are sleeping, but the impacts can be extreme. This can result in heart damage or death if left untreated.

- **Restless legs syndrome:** When you suffer from RLS, you have a sleep movement disorder. This causes you to feel like your legs are uncomfortable when you try to sleep, leading to you feeling the urge to move while attempting to fall asleep. In some cases, this can wake you up in the middle of the night as well, leading to struggles in staying asleep.

- **Narcolepsy:** When you suffer from narcolepsy, you feel extremely sleepy during the day and may even fall asleep at inopportune times suddenly and unexpectedly during the night. These people struggle to regulate their sleep-wake cycles, which leads to them feeling rested right after they wake up, but feeling sleepy throughout much of the day. Their sleep cycles are usually disjointed and not particularly restful.

Sleep Disorders and the Vagus Nerve

Due to the relationship between the vagus nerve and the parasympathetic nervous system, which is what regulates the rest-and-digest mode, an inactivation of the vagus nerve can cause an individual to struggle to sleep. Due to the heightened sympathetic response when the parasympathetic responses are muted, the individual will find themselves struggling to sleep well, all because the nerve that is supposed to regulate their ability to sleep fails to regulate itself.

Vagus nerve stimulation has been used to treat epilepsy, in which an implant electrically stimulates the vagus nerve. However, it has also been found to have a direct impact on the ability to regulate and has been linked to increased daytime alertness, meaning that the individual, especially if they are suffering from narcolepsy or something similar, will be able to stay awake longer.

The problem, however, is that it has been found that the vagus nerve stimulator, in particular the electrical stimulator, can cause an increase in apnea. This apnea can also worsen the occurrence rate of seizures in general, making it difficult to determine whether stimulating the vagus nerve electrically is a good fit for those struggling with sleep apnea or other sleep disorders.

Chapter 15: The Vagus Nerve and Epilepsy

Epilepsy is another common chronic disorder that people around the world suffer from. When someone suffers from epilepsy, they suffer from abnormal brain activity. This can cause periods of time in which they suffer from seizures or loss of consciousness. It is something that happens around the world, to people of all ages and backgrounds.

What is Epilepsy?

Epilepsy itself is a seizure disorder—it can vary greatly from person to person, but what is consistent is that the individual has abnormal brain activity. Seizures themselves can vary, and typically, those who have been diagnosed with epilepsy must have had at least two seizures that are confirmed before the diagnosis is given in the first place.

For some people, epilepsy can be treated with medication. For others, surgery can help manage the symptoms. Some people will age out of the seizures while others may suffer all their lives. Due to the complexity and variability of the brain, epilepsy does not present the same way in every person out there—it will vary based on the individual. That does not necessarily change the diagnosis—it just means that the treatment plan may vary.

Epilepsy Symptoms

Epilepsy is characterized primarily by abnormal brain activity of some sort. If you think of the brain as a computer for a moment, the seizure brought on by epilepsy would be the equivalent of your computer encountering an error and freezing up—it may crash completely, such as when your computer crashes and restarts, leading to the individual entirely losing consciousness. It may freeze up and stop responding for a moment—similar to an absence seizure. No matter the kind of seizure, however, there are several symptoms that are usually at least common. These symptoms include:

- **Confusion**
- **Staring**
- **Jerking or other movements that are entirely uncontrollable in the arms, legs, or entire body**
- **Losing consciousness entirely**
- **Emotional symptoms, such as extreme anxiety**

Seizures themselves happen and are relatively common—young children may have them during fevers during the first few years of life. Others may have them after a head injury, or others may just have the tendency to develop epilepsy due to genetics.

What is known, however, is that there are primarily six distinct forms of seizures: absence, tonic, atonic, clonic, myoclonic, and tonic-clonic seizures. Each of these will present differently and can appear entirely differently from the others.

- **Absence seizures:** These seizures are sometimes called "petit mal." They are noted as staring, sometimes believed to be daydreaming. However, when this happens, there is a brief malfunction of the brain and the individual temporarily loses awareness. These can happen one at a time, or in groups, known as clusters.
- **Tonic seizures:** These seizures lead to the individual suddenly going rigid—muscles are unconsciously stiffened, particularly in the torso, legs, and arms. Those who suffer from a tonic seizure may suddenly fall down if left to themselves
- **Atonic seizures:** Effectively, the opposite of tonic seizures: These lead to a drop to the ground and a lack of muscle control

- **Clonic seizures:** These seizures are rhythmic movements. This may be a constant twitch in the face or neck.

- **Myoclonic seizures:** These are sudden but short jerks of the arms or legs.

- **Tonic-clonic seizures:** These seizures are characterized by a sudden lack of consciousness, stiffening and jerking together, and sometimes, the individual may lose control of the bladder as well at the same time.

Epilepsy and the Vagus Nerve

Doctors and scientists are not yet sure how epilepsy and the vagus nerve are intricately related. What is known, however, is that shocking or stimulating the vagus nerve is an effective way to end a seizure in progress. Scientists noticed this connection in the 19th century, when they realized that sometimes, seizures would stop when pressure was applied to the carotid artery. As you may remember, the carotid artery and vagus nerve go together for a short period of time in the neck.

Over time, it was found that stimulating the nerve with electrical impulses would show a decrease in seizures in general. It is not necessarily immediate, but over time, through stimulation, the seizure activity slowed, and some people saw a cessation in seizures altogether.

When you are using vagus nerve stimulation to treat your epilepsy, you will have a small device implanted near your collarbone. It is then programmed to stimulate your vagus nerve at regular intervals, while also programmed to create a sudden burst of stimulation, which can be done with the use of a magnet to interrupt a seizure that is in progress at any given moment.

Despite the fact that scientists do not yet understand this link, it is undeniable—it does work to lessen seizure activity. Within a few months, around ¼ of people see that their seizure frequency has dropped in half. And after a year or two, upwards of 45% of people have found that the frequency of epileptic episodes has dropped by half. Of course, this treatment should never be taken instead of medication that has been prescribed by a doctor.

Chapter 16: The Vagus Nerve and Rheumatoid Arthritis

Rheumatoid arthritis is a disorder that falls into two different classifications that you have already seen thus far—it is an inflammatory autoimmune disorder. Remember, inflammatory disorders cause inflammation in the area, and the autoimmune disorder then attacks that particular area.

While some arthritis, namely osteoarthritis, is caused through simple wear-and-tear that is caused through overuse, rheumatoid arthritis is entirely self-inflicted—just not consciously. You cannot control that your body is attacking itself, and yet it continues to do so, sending the immune system after your joints or other body parts and attacking them. The lining in your joints can become weakened and painful, and you may even start to damage bone.

What is Rheumatoid Arthritis?

Rheumatoid arthritis can be broken down into two key words: Rheumatoid and arthritis. This offers you plenty of insight into what it is. Rheumatoid itself refers to inflammation or pain, particularly where it lingers in any sorts of joints or muscles.

Arthritis itself refers to any sort of joint inflammation. This makes rheumatoid arthritis almost redundant, but there is a reason for that—it is joint inflammation and pain that is literally caused by inflammation. The autoantibodies created by virtue of having an autoimmune disorder attack and inflame the joints, which then leads to arthritis to develop.

This is not a normal part of aging, and it something that is largely treatable, though not curable. It is particularly notable because it is largely symmetrical—it will occur on both sides of the body at the same time rather than developing due to wear on specific joints. However, rheumatoid arthritis does not stop at your joints: It can also impact the rest of your body—even in areas where there are no bones at all, such as the heart or lungs.

Rheumatoid Arthritis Symptoms

Rheumatoid arthritis has warning signs and symptoms that can cue you to making a point to investigate whatever is happening to you at that particular moment. When you suffer from rheumatoid arthritis, it may be easy to try to brush the pain off as being indicative of your aging, but remember, it is not a normal side effect of aging. Sure, you will feel slower and stiffer, but you should not have all of the inflammation and angry, red joints that go along with rheumatoid arthritis to begin with. Let's stop and take a look at the most common rheumatoid arthritis symptoms: Joint pain, stiffness, and fatigue.

Joint pain is usually characterized as either being slow-going or sudden in onset, depending on the individual. The individual will likely find that they have swollen joints that may look inflamed and red, meaning they are warm to the touch and also noticeably different. These joints can eventually disfigure if left untreated. The stiffness typically occurs first thing in the morning, or after a period of time in which you sat without moving for a while, such as if you work at a desk. You will feel stiff, and in some instances, like you cannot move at all. Fatigue is relatively straightforward—when you suffer from rheumatoid arthritis, you have a tendency to be exhausted sooner and longer than other people.

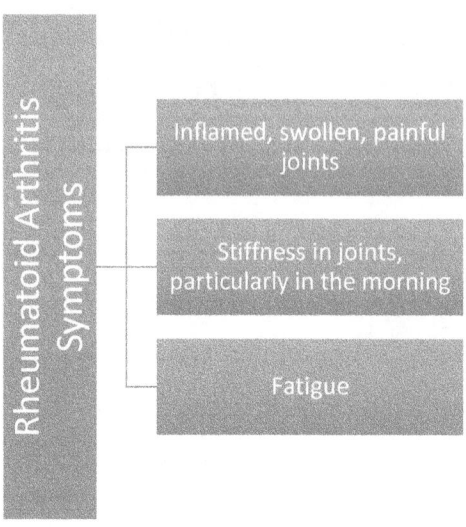

Rheumatoid Arthritis and the Vagus Nerve

By now, you should be pretty confident in your understanding of the link between the vagus nerve and inflammation and autoimmune disease. We have already established that the vagus nerve is responsible for sending the signals necessary to the brain to allow for the regulation of the immune system, which, when overstimulated or under-stimulated, can lead to a misfiring of the immune system, which can be particularly problematic for the individual suffering. This can cause either an immune system that is not functioning at all, or one that functions too well and attacks the body instead.

When you wish to treat your rheumatoid arthritis, then, you want to stimulate the vagus nerve, causing an inhibition of cytokine production, which should also reduce the inflammation associated with rheumatoid arthritis in the first place. There has been success using vagus nerve stimulators to create electrical impulses that travel directly to the vagus nerve, which then influences how the body is regulated. Those with rheumatoid arthritis who have attempted treatment in these manners have found that they show a massive improvement in their symptoms—they showed significant reduction in their DAS28-CRP scores, which is the measure of how active rheumatoid arthritis is at any given moment. Those pre-treatment were shown to have a 4.19, and after a week, they saw this number reduced down to 3.12, which shows mild activation of the disease at any given moment.

Effectively, then, you can use a vagus nerve stimulator to lessen the severity of your arthritis thanks to the anti-inflammatory effect of the stimulation in the first place. That reduction in symptoms can be significant, allowing for a massive improvement in quality of life that can be the difference between enjoying day-to-day activities and being entirely miserable in the first place.

Chapter 17: The Vagus Nerve and Other Symptoms

While thus far, the vagus nerve has been related to several autoimmune and other chronic illnesses, it is also related to other symptoms that can be problematic as well. This chapter will give you a brief overview of other symptoms that are directly influenced by the vagus nerve. As you read through these, if you feel like you are suffering from any of them yourself, it may be worth an attempt to use the natural vagus nerve stimulation methods that you will receive in Part III: Therapies and Exercises for Stimulating the Vagus Nerve, or speaking to your doctor. Remember, just because you are in pain does not mean that you are required to liver in misery or discomfort—you can absolutely make it a point to treat these symptoms and find a level of comfort that you are happy with.

The Vagus Nerve and Vasovagal Syncope

As the name itself implies, vasovagal syncope is directly related to your vagus nerve. When you suffer from one of these episodes, you will find yourself suddenly fainting. Usually, this is caused by an overreaction to a specific stimulus or distress. When you think of someone suddenly fainting in response to seeing blood, for example, that is the perfect example of a vasovagal syncope.

Essentially, when you suffer from one of these syncope episodes, you are exposed to some sort of stimulus that may be distressing to you. This could be bad news about yourself or someone else, or it could be the sight of something distressing, such as blood or an injury. In response, your vagus nerve shoots into overdrive—remember, its job is to regulate your stress response. In this instance, the vagus nerve overreacts, and because of that, you are flooded with a far higher dose of acetylcholine than intended. This, then, drops your blood pressure and heart rate significantly more than necessary, leading to you fainting. The sudden lack of blood flow to your brain due to the decreased blood pressure leads to the fainting spell.

This is harmless, but can be annoying, especially if it happens regularly or in response to something that you encounter regularly. If you do suffer from these episodes regularly, you may feel lightheaded leading up to the instance, or feel like you are suffering from tunnel vision. As this happens, the best way to prevent yourself from losing consciousness is to sit or lie down if you can and raise your legs above your head. This keeps the blood going to your brain instead of your legs, keeping you conscious.

The Vagus Nerve and Gastroparesis

Gastroparesis develops when your stomach becomes incapable of regulating itself, no longer being able to move food out of itself in a regular, normal amount of time. This is particularly common in people who have suffered from diabetes, but can be caused by other issues or injuries as well. When you have gastroparesis, the stomach muscles that are meant to contract to push food along become damaged or weak for some reason—this means that food lingers in your stomach instead of being pushed to the intestines for proper digestion. This, then, means that food gets stuck, where it can fester, rot, and lead to all sorts of other complications. You can get sick, you can suffer from nausea and heartburn, feel bloated, or even find yourself regularly vomiting up the food that you have eaten but not digested.

The nerve that is responsible for managing your stomach's muscles is the vagus nerve. When this nerve is damaged or just unresponsive for some particular reason, it can lead to these symptoms, in which the body is not moving food along, and that can be incredibly problematic—you can find that your appetite is all over the place, or that your blood sugar is crashing due to never digesting food.

This, of course, has other complications as well: if the food does not actually rot and ferment, causing digestive issues, it can instead become a bezoar—a solid blockage that will prevent food from passing through, even if the muscle becomes active again. It can even cause malnutrition or blood sugar issues, particularly if the food stays stuck in the stomach and then suddenly dumps all at once into the intestines, suddenly spiking blood sugar.

Other Vagus Nerve Related Issues

There are other issues that a vagus nerve that is dysfunctional in some way can trigger as well, such as the following:

- **Nausea—especially chronically**

- **Unintended weight loss:** this is usually in tandem with nausea

- **Weight gain:** When you are depressed and chronically fatigued, you may struggle to exercise regularly, leading to weight gain

- **Heart rate regulation issues:** This can manifest as both bradycardia (heart rate too slow) or tachycardia (heart rate too quick)

- **Irritable bowel syndrome:** Due to muscles not moving properly or due to autoimmune issues, the bowels can find themselves inflamed and uncomfortable—potentially compounding with weight loss when nothing is comfortable to eat

- **Depression:** All the feeling ill can lead to some pretty low moods

- **Heartburn:** This usually comes along with gastroparesis—when the stomach is not regulating properly, you are going to be uncomfortable. In this case, the esophageal sphincter remains open, allowing acid to splash up (reflux)

- **Dizziness:** You may not always faint, but dizziness can also be related to the vagus nerve running haywire for similar reasons to the syncope episodes

Part III
Therapies and Exercises for Stimulating the Vagus Nerve

Chapter 18: Vagus Nerve Stimulation

Vagus nerve stimulation is particularly promising in the treatment for several of the complications you have read about thus far, and that effectiveness has been briefly touched upon in several of the previous chapters. Nevertheless, this chapter will provide you with a brief understanding of what vagus nerve stimulation is.

As you know now, the vagus nerve is largely responsible for the regulation between the body and mind—it allows you to regulate what is happening in your entire body. It is effectively responsible for maintaining homeostasis within your body, which is primarily what allows your body to function as intended. However, for some people the vagus nerve can get out of whack somehow—for some, it may be due to injury or as a complication of an unrelated illness, such as diabetic neuropathy. Despite how easily damaged and fragile the vagus nerve may be, it is incredibly important. Without it, your body will struggle to regulate itself properly.

Electrical (Direct) Vagus Nerve Stimulation

This is where vagus nerve stimulation comes in. In recent years, thanks to all sorts of recent medical advancements, you can now directly stimulate your vagus nerve through an implanted device. This is perfect, if your body needs this sort of literal shock to regulate itself. As you have seen, this can be fantastic for treating epilepsy, for example. This stimulation can help you in several ways, such as stopping your body from producing inflammatory cytokines, or in regulating how quickly or slowly your heart beats. However, electrical stimulation also have several side effects as well.

When treating epilepsy with a vagus nerve stimulator, there are several potential side effects. Some of them are annoying, but tolerable, while others may be incredibly harmful to the individual. One of the side effects listed for the VNS is cardiac death, which of course, is a terrifying thought to face if you are considering this implant for yourself. Beyond that, there are several other side effects listed:

- **Bradycardia**
- **Nausea**
- **Struggling to swallow**

- **Changes to the voice**
- **Hoarseness and coughing**
- **Shortness of breath**
- **Discomfort, pain, or tingling**
- **Headaches**
- **Sleepiness**
- **Sleep apneas**

For someone seriously considering this treatment, these symptoms and side effects can be enough to entirely forego this treatment altogether. That is, of course, always an option for you. Just because a doctor has recommended one of these devices does not mean that you have to opt to have it implanted. This is not the only way to trigger the vagus nerve either—there are several methods that you can use to naturally trigger the vagus nerve as well.

Natural Vagus Nerve Stimulation

When you choose to stimulate your vagus nerve yourself, through natural means, you are avoiding the electric shocks to your nerve altogether, and saving yourself from undergoing surgery. Do keep in mind that perhaps one of the greatest differences between using a medical device and choosing to stimulate your nerve yourself is that in triggering your own vagus nerve is far more difficult to regulate. This is not necessarily bad—it just means that you are not going to get as precise or as regular a result as you otherwise would have gotten through direct, programmed machinery dosing you at regular intervals.

On the other hand, however, you also do not find yourself suffering from any of the side effects or having to recover from a surgery either. When you choose to trigger your vagus nerve through natural means, you are essentially tapping into the fact that the vagus nerve is intertwined with the vast majority of your body. You can then effectively stimulate specific areas of your body in certain ways in order to send the necessary feedback to your vagus nerve, pushing it into using parasympathetic processes rather than allowing for the continuance of the sympathetic ones that you are likely trying to rein in when using one of these methods.

Beyond the overview of the electrical device, this book will primarily look at ways that you can activate and stimulate your vagus nerve on your own. You will learn several different methods to tap into your vagus nerve, using your own personal, built in process that is there for you to trigger yourself to calm down or regulate your body. As you learn these processes, you can force yourself to calm down. If you are having an anxiety attack? You can trigger those parasympathetic reflexes with ease, leading to your entire body calming down. Do you suffer from a sleep disorder, such as insomnia? Using these processes, you can relax your body and shift yourself into parasympathetic rest-and-digest mode in minutes. Do you suffer from inflammation? Perhaps a yoga regimen that activates your vagus nerve can help you. Keep in mind that as you go through these methods, they are not meant to override the opinion of a doctor that has examined you and your file—this book is not a replacement for proper medical advice by a proper medical professional in front of you.

Chapter 19: Breathing to Stimulate the Vagus Nerve

When you are frightened, have you ever noticed how your breathing picks up? This is in response to your sympathetic nervous system—your body is literally being pushed into fight-flight-freeze mode in preparation to keep itself alive. When you wish to calm yourself down from those feelings of panic, you may unconsciously put yourself through deep breathing exercises in an attempt to regulate yourself. Do you know why?

Most people do not realize it, but those deep breaths actually are triggering to your vagus nerve that it is time to get to work. The vagus nerve is essentially goaded into acting in a way that will allow for the alleviation of symptoms and slowing of the heart rate because the vagus nerve activates the parasympathetic nervous system.

Without the vagus nerve and this little feedback loop, your heart rate would likely sit around 100 bpm naturally. It would rarely drop lower, and your heart rate would be free to skyrocket without limitation, which of course, could be dangerous. The parasympathetic nervous system keeps that from happening—the parasympathetic system's purpose is essentially to put the brakes on the sympathetic nervous system. It is the regulator—

the part of you that is able to calm you down and convince you to relax. It slows your heart rate and helps you achieve that state of calm that you may be looking for after an anxiety attack.

Breathing and the Vagus Nerve: How it Works

When you are breathing, have you ever noticed how your heart rate changes? When you take in a deep breath, you may feel your pulse quicken, and as you exhale, you notice it drop again. This is for a very specific reason—your vagus nerve is regulating your heart rate. When you breathe in, you trigger your pulse to quicken, and as your pulse quickens, it raises blood pressure.

That raise in blood pressure and pulse triggers your parasympathetic nervous system to kick in—it wants to regulate your heart rate, so it dumps some acetylcholine into your blood stream, slowing the heart rate. This is important to keep in mind—it means that you can effectively kick your vagus nerve into action simply by taking a deep breath in and cuing to the nerve that you are in need of some regulation to keep your heart rate steady. Your vagus nerve, as you exhale, is at its most active, slowing your heart rate the most. This means, then, that you are able to effectively regulate yourself and your parasympathetic nervous system all through breathing.

This is nothing new—in fact, the breathing pattern that triggers this state of calmness thanks to the parasympathetic nervous system actually arises in several different calming, spiritual activities. Mantras used during any sort of meditation can trigger this sort of activation, creating the proper timing between breaths and holding them, as do saying the Ave Maria prayer. The breathing rate during these techniques is dropped down to about six breaths every minute, which is what these breathing techniques will aim for.

Valsalva Maneuver

The first breathing technique that you will look at to trigger the parasympathetic response you are looking for is the Valsalva maneuver. This technique can aid in identifying how one's heart works, particularly with the autonomic nervous system. When you use this method, keep in mind that for those with heart issues already, you should ask a doctor before attempting this process. It does put a strain at the heart while also triggering a regulation of the heart rate.

You will primarily fall back on this method if you find that your heart rate is too high, such as during a panic attack. When used properly, you will find that your body will regulate itself out, allowing you to slow your breathing and regulate yourself better.

This process involves four phases that you go through with a series of five steps.

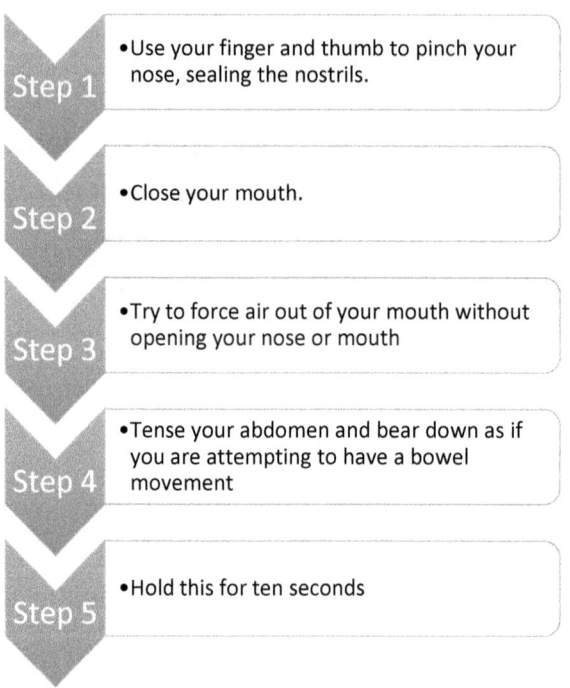

- **Step 1**: Use your finger and thumb to pinch your nose, sealing the nostrils.
- **Step 2**: Close your mouth.
- **Step 3**: Try to force air out of your mouth without opening your nose or mouth
- **Step 4**: Tense your abdomen and bear down as if you are attempting to have a bowel movement
- **Step 5**: Hold this for ten seconds

These five steps take you through four different physiological stages that are effectively able to regulate your body. As you go through each and every one of these stages, you will find yourself feeling better and more regulated. These phases are:

- **Phase 1:** You create pressure within your chest due to blowing against closed airways while simultaneously bearing down. When you do this, blood is forced to the limbs, creating a spike in blood pressure.

- **Phase 2:** You cause your blood pressure to drop as blood from the veins returns to the heart. The autonomic nervous system senses this drop and then raises your heart rate, returning your blood pressure to healthy ranges.

- **Phase 3:** You relax and let go of the breath and pressure you have created. This triggers a drop in blood pressure again.

- **Phase 4:** As blood returns to your heart, blood flow will return to normal, but blood pressure will rise in response to the constricted blood vessels, and then blood pressure causes the heart rate to return to normal as well.

Diaphragmatic Breathing

When you use diaphragmatic breathing, you are looking to trigger your body to relax. This sort of breathing can lead to a decrease in your stress, heart rate, and allow for the regulation of your vagus nerve's stimulation. When you are using diaphragmatic breathing, you are effectively using breathing exercises that directly engage with the diaphragm, the muscle in your abdomen responsible for controlling your breathing.

To begin this process, find an area in which you can be comfortable. Start somewhere that you will be comfortable in, sitting, standing, or lying down. You may choose to stretch on the floor or a bed, or sit on a chair that you are comfortable on. With your position that you are comfortable in identified, relax your shoulders.

As your shoulders fall and relax, put one hand on your chest and another on your stomach. Breathe in through your nose as you do this for roughly two seconds, noticing how the air expands your stomach. You want to make sure your chest remains still as you breathe in—this is how you know that you are using your diaphragm to breathe instead of your chest, which is not going to be as deep or relaxing.

With your lips pursed, as if you were trying to take a sip with a straw or water bottle, press down on your stomach to remind yourself to breathe out with the abdomen and exhale for two seconds. You will repeat this process over and over, and as you do, start to stretch the time for the inhale and exhale up to five seconds each. This will regulate your breathing to 6 breaths per minute, which is the sort of vagus nerve activation sweet spot.

Chapter 20: Temperature to Stimulate the Vagus Nerve

Another technique that you can use to stimulate your vagus nerve is to trigger a shift in temperature. In particular, when you suddenly expose yourself to the cold, you can stimulate your vagus nerve. Now, taking a cold shower or dipping yourself into a winter lake may not sound particularly pleasant, and you may not enjoy the process, but the end result is undeniable—you activate your vagus nerve, which then, of course, activates parasympathetic activity, allowing you to then regulate your body

How it Works

As you cool yourself off, exposing yourself to sudden acute cold, you are able to cause several different effects—you are able to speed up the metabolism while also causing any swelling, inflammation, or other discomfort to lessen. This is exactly why you are told to put ice on a swollen or otherwise inflamed part of your body—the ice alleviates the swelling. The exposure to the cold can also increase the rest that you get, allowing your sleep to improve in quality, which is why many people in northern countries have a tendency to leave their children sleeping on a cold winter day.

When you want to do this for yourself, you effectively trigger your body to constrict the blood vessels, just like you did in the Valsalva maneuver, which then enables the body to start regulating itself. Beyond the myriad of other benefits, you will trigger your heart rate to slow down through exposing yourself to the cold for a short period of time.

Of course, this does not mean you should go play in the snow for an extended period of time without any proper winter gear. It is always important to remember to take care of yourself—make sure that you are warm enough and regulating yourself when you are making it a point to use this method, otherwise you run serious health risks, such as hypothermia or frostbite. Nevertheless, short, acute exposures to this sort of sudden drop of temperature can do wonders to regulate your vagus nerve's activation. Of course, there are several different ways that you can activate your vagus nerve through exposure to the cold.

Ice Baths

One such way is through ice baths—this is often seen by athletes, especially after a long workout session. In this, you are doing exactly what it sounds like—you are bathing in ice water. You may do this in an icy cold swimming pool or bathtub, for example, or you may even go through the process of dipping yourself into an icy cold river or lake on a winter day. No matter how you go through this process, remember that you are doing so for a brief period—you do not want to inflict harm, but rather go through the cold long enough to reap the benefits.

When you do this, you will see several benefits—you will find yourself feeling far more awake, thanks to the sudden shock to your system. This will also make you take deeper breaths, which activates your vagus nerve as already discussed. As you do this as well, you will see that you willpower increases—while this may not necessarily be directly related to any of the illnesses that have been discussed thus far, it is still a pretty cool benefit! You may even see weight loss as your body makes it a point to create brown fat instead of the usual fat that is developed. Brown fat is the fat that infants have naturally—it is a massive user of energy, which allows for the extra burning of calories.

Cryo Therapy

Another method that has grown popular lately that may be a bit less accessible to you but is still legitimate nevertheless is through cryo therapy. This involves you standing in a small, enclosed space and being blasted with cold air. Think of this as an air conditioner in a small space on steroids—it is meant to be extreme cold for a short period of time. This may not help you if you are not in an area where this is an option, or if you are unwilling or unable to spend the money that such a therapy would cost, but it has still become popular.

Splashing Cold Water on Face

The most accessible of the options, especially year-round, is through using cold water that you splash on your face when you feel like you need to calm down or self-regulate. If you feel overly emotional, as if you are panicking or anxious, or generally just out of sorts, try splashing cold water on your face or taking a quick cold shower. Doing so triggers the same effect as the previous methods, but it is free and easily accessible, no matter where you are. You can even go through this process out and about, simply by entering a restroom and using their sink for a moment to cool yourself off before continuing on with your day.

Chapter 21: Singing to Stimulate the Vagus Nerve

Have you ever wondered why so many people, when they meditate, seem to moan? In fact, if you heard meditation as a concept, was your first thought to think of someone sitting, cross-legged and saying, "OM" in a really deep voice? This is for a good reason—that sort of noise directly stimulates the vagus nerve. While it most likely was not understood at the time how this sort of movement and sound would directly impact the individuals and why these sort of chants and hums would trigger such a state of calm, it has been found to do so.

This is because it triggers the vagus nerve, and as you trigger the vagus nerve, you encourage your body to go into a parasympathetic state instead of allowing the sympathetic responses to rule your body. As you learn to take back that control, learning how to activate your vagus nerve on a whim, you can force yourself into feeling calmer, even if you were in the middle of an anxiety attack just moments earlier.

How it Works

When you sing, or hum or chant or do anything else that makes sound at the back of your throat, you are using your vocal cords. These cords tie into the vagus nerve—or rather, the vagus nerve ties around them, and as you make these deep, low, guttural sounds, you are actively stimulating your vagus nerve, almost directly. As you do so, you are essentially exercising your vagus nerve, allowing yourself to increase the tone of your nerve, which can then enable you to better regulate yourself.

As you are stimulating the vagus nerve, you activate it, and as you activate it, you create the effect of calming yourself down. Your nerve communicates to your brain that it has been stimulated and therefore it is time for the body to relax and calm down. This is exactly why these sorts of sounds are so frequently used in meditation, yoga, and other forms of movement and mindfulness that are meant to control your ability to calm yourself down.

Further, as you go through this process through humming or singing, you are forcing yourself to manage your breathing. As you do so, you are activating your vagus nerve in yet another way as well. This may not be the most practical of methods, as there are plenty of situations in which singing to yourself is not necessarily going to be welcomed—you cannot just burst into song during your next job interview or while you are stressing out as you walk down the street. Well, you can, but your results will probably not be what you were hoping for!

However, this can be used when you are on your own. If you are awake late at night and struggling to sleep, for example, you may be able to sing to yourself in order to trigger yourself to start to calm down. If you are in your car driving down the freeway and stressed out because you are, you can always try singing as well.

How to Use Sounds to Activate Vagus Nerve

When you want to use these processes to activate your own vagus nerve, you want to think big, low, and guttural. The deeper the sound, the more likely it is that your vocal cord's movements and vibrations will penetrate the vagus nerve, and the more likely it is that your breathing will be regulated properly to get the right effect. This means that if you wish to do so, you can try singing along to a song that you know is lower and throatier, for example, Adele sings plenty of songs that would engage the notes necessary for this process.

When in doubt or when you do not have a song in mind, you can simply hum to yourself. All you need to do is make sure that your note is deep, loud, and consistent. When you do this, do not worry about embarrassing yourself or trying to be perfect—you are not attempting to become a rock star; you are attempting to regulate your vagus nerve, which is entirely unrelated. You do not have to be good to get the desired effects or to ensure that you are comfortable—all you need to do is make sure that you trigger the right part of your anatomy to get the desired result.

Chapter 22: Coffee Enema to Stimulate the Vagus Nerve

For some people, the word enema may be enough to skip this chapter altogether, and that is okay! You have several other options available to you at this point. However, for those of you who are either morbidly curious or legitimately interested in going through this process, keep reading—you are about to learn all about how a coffee enema—yes, injecting coffee into your colon—can help you stimulate your vagus nerve. Despite how strange this may sound, this is a fantastic way to stimulate your vagus nerve.

The Gut-Brain Axis:

This process works because the vagus nerve works from the brain to the gut and back again—it does an entire loop. This means that you can have the brain communicating with the gut while the gut is simultaneously communicating with the brain. This is what the vagus nerve facilitates—it allows for that communicate easily and effectively. This allows for the vagus nerve to control how the body digests food and the blood flow necessary to go through digestion altogether. When that is not working, when there is poor communication between the brain and gut, you run into several of the issues that have already been discussed thus far in the book. Digestion slows or stops, constipation or IBS develops, and the individual suffering probably feels miserable. This gut-brain axis means that you can tell when there is something wrong with the gut because of the state of the brain and vice-versa. This means, then, if you can stimulate the vagus nerve, you can effectively start to fix the problems you are seeing described here. This is where the coffee enema comes in

How the Coffee Enema Works

When you seek to use the vagus nerve through a coffee enema, you are effectively forcing the point of stimulation of the neurons within the guts. Just as how your muscles will atrophy when you cannot use them, your nerves struggle to function after going unused for an extended period of time. They start to lose their ability to function. This is what the coffee enema is addressing—when you are using a coffee enema, you are effectively triggering the nerve pathways within the colon to begin communicating with the vagus nerve and therefore the brain again.

This works primarily because the colon's job is to absorb the liquid that is within your waste—this keeps you from constantly excreting water that your body otherwise needs to stay hydrated. When you use a coffee enema, then, you are triggering the absorption of liquid into your colon. There are two key acids that are present in coffee that are important. These are kahweol and cafestol palmitate. Your colon absorbs these, and as it does so, the acids boost the production of the enzymes in the liver by upwards of 700%.

When you trigger these enzymes, you then trigger a detoxification process—the enzyme produced then binds to any of the toxins within the liver and then excretes the waste. Considering how frequently the body's blood supply circulates through the liver, once every three minutes, you can effectively filter out your blood incredibly quickly.

Through the use of these enemas, you will start to see all sorts of regulation—you will see that bowel function and digestion starts to improve as the nerves are reactivated and strengthened. Of course, if you are sensitive to caffeine, you may be a bit wary about this process. However, the enema process does not cause much of the caffeine to be absorbed in the first place. The body does not naturally absorb caffeine through the colon, and you are likely to absorb 3.5x less caffeine through an enema that you would otherwise ingest drinking the coffee.

Using a Coffee Enema

When you want to perform a coffee enema, you want to make sure that you set aside an hour for the process. Try to make sure that you will be entirely uninterrupted during this process and make your bathroom as comfortable as possible for the process. You will be in there the entire time in order to minimize mess and make the process as simple as possible. This process will have several steps that you will go through.

Step 1: Prep the coffee

At this point, you want to make coffee—preferably organic and freshly ground by you right before use for the best effect. As a beginner, start with brewing coffee with ½ teaspoon of grounds. You can increase the number over time, but starting low is in your best interest. From there, mix the grounds with filtered water and boil the coffee for 10 minutes before straining it.

Make sure now that you allow the coffee to cool. It should reach room temperature. Resist the urge to simply place the coffee in the fridge or throw some ice into it—your colon is incredibly sensitive when it comes to temperature, and the closer to room temperature you can get it, the better. As a general rule of thumb, make sure that you can tolerate comfortably touching the liquid coffee for at least five seconds with the temperature you are going to use.

Step 2: The enema

Now, this stage can be intimidating. You will want to do this in the bathroom, preferably in a bathtub just in case you have any accidents since you will not be used to holding the enema at first. If you cannot do this, set up several towels underneath you on the bathroom floor. Fill the enema bag with coffee and release the air that is trapped within the closed bag.

Now, you will want to make sure that the bag is situated above you a few feet to allow gravity to do its job while the hose can reach you. Lubricate the hose's tip with either a personal lubricant or even olive or coconut oil if you do not have any at the moment. Lay down on your right side and tuck your knees in toward your abdomen before inserting the hose's tip within the rectum. Slowly allow the coffee to drain in. Remember, this will not necessarily be comfortable the first time, but should not be painful. If you are cramping, stop for a moment until it passes and then allow for the flow of liquid again. As you do this, allow as much as you are comfortable with.

With the coffee inserted, lay in position for two minutes before rotating to your back for two more minutes. If you can, hold the liquid for anywhere between 5 and 15 minutes, but do not force it if you are uncomfortable. When the time is up or you are no longer comfortable, it is okay to release into the toilet.

At that point, follow the cleaning instructions on your enema kit before putting everything away. Doing this may leave you feeling as if you have a headache or tired, though this could be because you have just released toxins from your body. Make it a point to stay hydrated afterwards for best results.

Chapter 23: Mindfulness to Stimulate the Vagus Nerve

Mindfulness is a process through which you become aware of your body, relaxing deeply and allowing your body to go through its thought processes without interruption or influence. When you go through mindfulness, you are effectively meditating, and doing so can have fantastic results on your mental health. This sort of meditation can directly influence your state of mind, helping to cope with depression and anxiety. It can make you happier and more able to focus and function. It can help people cope with pain. It has also been shown to reduce the biomarkers for inflammation.

Now, compare those effects of mindfulness to those that you have learned about thus far through learning about the vagus nerve—they are incredibly similar. Thanks to how similar they are, what happens the two are connected together?

The answer is that you get increased results. You are able to remain calm while also getting all of the fantastic benefits of stimulating the vagus nerve in the first place. The best way to do this, then, is to utilize vagus nerve stimulation into your mindfulness routine. If you do not have a mindfulness routine already, this chapter will give you one to follow while still utilizing vagus nerve activation.

How it Works

Mindfulness allows for the individual to essentially detach from emotions, pain, or anything else that is actively occurring at that moment that is unpleasant or uncomfortable. This means, then, that the individual can better cope with any discomfort. In coping better, the individual can then manage their ability to relax and cope, effectively ensuring that they are able to regulate their heart rate.

Through breathing techniques during mindfulness, you take control of your physical self. This allows you to take deep breaths and directly impact your vagus nerve and therefore heart rate. Doing so then enables you to better regulate, and that is likely where some of the anti-inflammatory benefits of mindfulness come into play. However, this chapter will have you combine a mindfulness technique with a technique you have already learned—using your voice to activate the vagus nerve. This will create a compounded effect in which you are able to better trigger the vagus nerve and create a better effect overall.

Using Mindfulness

When you are utilizing mindfulness, you are effectively teaching yourself to pay attention to the moment that you are in right then. You are entirely accepting what is happening around you and because of that, you are able to better regulate your own emotional response. You are willing to accept exactly what is going on, and because of that acceptance, you can then calm yourself down and focus on your breathing. As you do, you find that you are far more capable of coping with whatever is happening around you in the first place. Most often, these techniques go hand-in-hand with coping with stress or anxiety, both of which the vagus nerve can help manage.

In order to begin, start by sitting down somewhere that you know you will be comfortable and where you can remain relatively uninterrupted. Straighten out your back, allow your feet to rest on the floor and place your hands onto your legs. Your arms and shoulders should be relaxed, though your back must remain straight at this point. You can keep your eyes opened or closed, depending on your own comfort. Whatever you prefer is fine, so long as you are not being distracted by the world around you.

Now, take a moment to pull in a deep breath. You should inhale deeply through your nose, feeling the air travel through your body and to your lungs. Make the breath long and slow, preferably five seconds as you do so. Hold it for a moment before exhaling out of your mouth. Make a low, deep hum as you do so—you could do the stereotypical "Om" sound or simply hum to yourself, depending on your comfort. Allow the hum to last another five seconds as you breathe through your mouth. You will repeat this process, preferably for ten to fifteen minutes if you can manage it. At first, even just five minutes may seem like a struggle, and that is okay. This process takes practice.

When you are going through this process, you may notice that your thoughts are wandering. Make a quick note of whatever your thoughts went to and then gently redirect your thoughts back to your breathing and humming. Getting distracted is normal from time to time, especially when you are new to the process in general. Instead of worrying about it, instead just focus on your breathing and how you are feeling with every inhale and exhale.

Try to go through this process relatively regularly—once or twice a day is a fantastic beginning point, especially as you are working to tone your vagus nerve and as the times that you can focus are shorter. These practices should be used as frequently as you may find them useful, or as often as you would like to.

When you use these processes, you will find yourself returning to a state of calm or relaxation, and that should be enough of a reinforcement that going through this process should quickly be enjoyable and calming. What is important, especially at first, however, is regularity. You want to do this at least daily, even if only for a few quick moments first thing in the morning. Even a little mindfulness is better than no mindfulness!

Chapter 24: Movement to Stimulate the Vagus Nerve

When you are using movement in order to stimulate the vagus nerve, you are effectively teaching your vagus nerve to become more flexible. Yoga in particular has been found to be incredibly effective at increasing your vagal tone, which would then create all of the desired effects that have been discussed thus far in the book. As you are able to better your vagal tone, you should start to notice that your body is more likely to be highly and fully functional, enabling you to start seeing relief.

The movements that you will discuss within this chapter will help you develop the tone that you will need to activate those parasympathetic pathways wherever and whenever you need them. As you learn to switch between the systems at will, you will find yourself happier, calmer, and likely feeling healthier as well. Remember, each of these movements will stimulate the vagus nerve in some way—they may directly stimulate it or indirectly stimulate it, but the end result is still the same: A more toned nerve that is more capable of handling anything life happens to throw its way.

The Half-Smile and the Vagus Nerve

The vagus nerve travels throughout the jaw and throat—it has to in order to regulate speech, sensation in the mouth, and taste. This means, then, that if you can start a half-smile, you can directly communicate with the vagus nerve. This process is simple enough to go through and with practice, you will start to activate your parasympathetic nervous system.

Stop and think about your face for a moment. Take a deep breath before relaxing the muscles that you associate with your expressions—namely, your cheeks and lips. As you do this, imagine that you are allowing your jaw to hang and relax while also gently and subtly pulling your lips back into a half smile. This is usually referred to as the social nervous system, which is yet another branch off the vagus nerve that is responsible for regulating your responses to other people.

While you smile, stop and envision your body, melting the tension away from yourself and letting relaxation flood over you. Imagine it pouring over you gently from the top of your head and pay attention to the way that it makes you feel as you do so. You should start to feel more relaxed, at ease, and willing to go through with your day.

Expanding and Opening the Chest

This method opens and stimulates the vagus nerve through stretching out your chest, opening it up and engaging with the vagus nerve indirectly. When you wish to use this technique, start by sitting down and place your hands onto your shoulders. This may be awkward, but it will be important. Take a deep breath, and as you do so, push your elbows inwards until they touch in front of you, and exhale as you touch your chin. Follow this process several times, inhaling as you first expand your chest, and exhale as you are pressing your elbows together. With a few quick repetitions of this process, you will find yourself feeling far better in no time at all.

Yoga—Child's Pose

Yoga itself is incredibly effective in helping your relax and activate your parasympathetic nervous system. When you are using this, you are combining yoga, breathing, and mindfulness to relax and meditate for a moment, allowing you to clear your mind while also activating that parasympathetic response that stimulates the vagus nerve.

One such pose you can use to do so is child's pose—this will involve you making sure your knees are spread as widely as possible on the floor while you sink your stomach down to the floor, between the thighs. Your feet should be flat on the ground, toes pointing behind you and tucked underneath your bottom. Your forehead will touch the floor and you will stretch your arms out as far as possible.

Within this pose, you will be stretching out all of the important nerves that are directly involved in the vagus nerve and its stimulation, allowing you to activate it, and you will also find that your stretching is comfortable and relaxing as well. Doing so enables you to start to activate those nerves and see the benefits.

When you sink into this position, remain for as long as you are comfortable—some people will enjoy it far longer than others. The important part here is to stretch gently to help yourself feel better. It is not designed to hurt. If you need to make any modifications, such as not stretching your knees out or not pressing your torso to the floor that is okay too. All that matters is you are stretching out within a similar pose in order to see the benefits. If you are not yet flexible enough or uncomfortable, modify the pose in any way that can help you reach that more comfortable position.

Chapter 25: Balancing the Gut Microbiome to Heal the Vagus Nerve

Remember, the gut and the vagus nerve are intricately linked—we have already looked at this repeatedly. This means, then, that you should also be able to heal the vagus nerve and your parasympathetic response through the gut. You see this often in people attempting to treat mental health issues—they will often change up their diet to something healthier in order to ensure that they are as healthy and effective as possible. After all, the gut communicates to the brain, so much so that the gut is often referred to as a second brain. Your gut will control your behavior thanks to the bacteria within the system.

This means, then, that it is crucial to ensure that the gut microbiome you have is as healthy as possible. This chapter will provide you with a handful of tips to balance your own gut microbiome. As you do so, you should find that your digestive system functions better, and as it functions better, your vagus nerve should also begin to function better as a result, thanks to just how closely they are linked to each other.

Plan for Plants

Plant-based diets are important—they create plenty of fiber that will help regulate your digestive system. This food gets passed through the system entirely undigested until the colon, at which point the bacteria should start to break it down. It will be able to break down much of the fiber through fermentation and unlocking polysaccharides. As it does so, it turns them into fatty acids, which is used for energy. This helps the cells within your colon, providing them the energy that is needed to keep the whole system running effectively.

Of course, it is also important to keep in mind that the fiber will also keep all of the food moving within your system as well. With enough fiber, issues with constipation or diarrhea should cease.

Fermented Foods

Fermented foods may have strong tastes that may be off-putting at first, but if you can develop a taste for them, these foods are fantastic for you. They include all sorts of bacteria that is actually healthy for your gut, and the more healthy bacteria is present within your gut, the less room there is for any bad, unhealthy bacteria that is going to cause you problems in the long run. If you can make it a point to eat some of these fermented foods, then, you should be able to get that gut balance back in order.

When you are eating fermented foods, you want to aim for eating it at least once, but preferably twice, a day. This can include foods such as tempeh or miso, while other people prefer kimchi for a quick, spicy bite, and others prefer a scoop of sauerkraut tossed onto a sausage. No matter what your flavor preference, spicy, savory, or otherwise, you should be able to find something for you.

Polyphenol

This is a micronutrient that behaves as an antioxidant. When you consume antioxidants, you are able to decrease inflammation in the body, allowing for the healing and managing of several of the illnesses and diseases discussed within this book. The antioxidant properties also allow the bacteria that is beneficial to flourish while helping you wipe out the bad bacteria that will only serve to cause you problems in the future.

You can find polyphenol in several foods that you may actually be thrilled to see have made the cut in healing your gut biome: Dark chocolate and red wine are two fantastic sources that are high in polyphenol. Other sources include blueberries, cherries, and green tea. Essentially, you want to ramp up the antioxidants.

Prebiotics are Your Friend

Foods that are rich in prebiotics essentially feed the good bacteria in your gut. The prebiotics are fibers that you cannot digest, but the bacteria will, and if you flood your body with these prebiotics, consuming them on the regular, you will find that the body is more able to keep that balance of good bacteria you need.

There are several foods that are rich in these prebiotics, such as bananas that are not yet ripe, oatmeal, rice or potatoes that have been cooked, then cooled, to allow the starches to resettle, and even onion and garlic. While your breath and your friends in person may not thank you for eating your daily dose of garlic and onion, your gut bacteria will be thrilled.

Probiotics are Your (Other) Friend

Along with the prebiotics that you are ingesting, you also want to fill in a probiotic as well. When you ingest probiotics, you are able to effectively plant the bacteria that you need to support the good gut bacteria in your digestive tract. When you use probiotics, you are effectively reintroducing those good bacteria into your gut, planting the foundation they will need to flourish and take over, then enabling you to heal your gut effectively.

When you are buying probiotics, you want to aim for those that are high in Lactobacillus and Bifidobacterium. particularly those that fall into a class known as soil-based organisms. These are more likely to make it through the digestive system alive and intact, allowing it to grow properly. You also want to make sure that whichever source you choose is high in diversity.

Bye-bye, Sugar!

Sugar is doing you no favors. The only bacteria that actually enjoy artificial and added refined sugars are the bad bacteria. Of course, these will also convince you that you need more of it to get through your day, leading to you feeling cravings for sugary food while simultaneously leaving you feeling miserable as a result. It is better just to cut out the added sugars altogether.

Look out for Antibiotics

Of course, it is impossible to avoid antibiotics all of the time. They can be necessary sometimes, particularly if you are sick or get an infection. When this happens, try to be proactive to protect as much of your good gut flora as possible. When you take any antibiotics, try to make sure that they are taken in tandem with antibiotic-resistant forms of yeast along with prebiotics and probiotics. The hope will be to keep the good bacteria populating the guts, even if it is still being wiped out with every dose of your antibiotic that you take. By protecting the gut while keeping it full of good bacteria between your antibiotics, you can reduce some of the strain and discomfort that will naturally go along with killing off your gut bacteria in the first place, such as diarrhea and nausea.

Conclusion

Thank you for making it through to the end of *Vagus Nerve*. Hopefully, you found this process to be informative and useful to you. It was intended to be a guide to learning all about the vagus nerve, how to recognize problems that may arise when the vagus nerve is struggling to function effectively, and then how best to manage any distress that goes along with the vagus nerve malfunction in the first place. As you read through this book, hopefully you found some information that was insightful, beneficial to you, and useful to use.

Within this book, you were introduced to several different concepts, ranging from the vagus nerve even existing to the mind-gut axis, the several systems that the nervous system is responsible for, and more. You were walked through exactly how to understand the sympathetic and parasympathetic nervous system, learning how the two are closely linked and responsible for managing so much of the body's reactions to the world at large. You learned all about how the vagus nerve regulates these processes, acting as a sort of mediator between the two so neither gets out of hand or hurts you.

Unfortunately, however, sometimes the nerve is off somehow. It can be over or under-active, and either of those can lead to serious problems for the individual suffering. This is where *Vagus Nerve* came in. You were taught several ways that you could activate your vagus nerve at home, some of which were conventional and others a bit less so. Nevertheless, with the several methods provided, you were given several options and ideas through which you could activate your own vagus nerve to help your own health improve for the better. Through stimulating your vagus nerve, you should start to see physical and mental health benefits.

From here, you must choose what you would like to do next. If you are interested in learning more about the biopsychology of the vagus nerve, that is one option for you—you could make it a point to study the interaction between the various nervous systems, learning more about exactly how that one (not-so-) little nerve is able to interact with your entire body, uniting a mind and a body together into one cohesive force.

If you wish to discuss getting a vagus nerve stimulator implanted, you can move forward with discussing that process with your doctor to discover if that is an option for you in the first place. You can see if that is a valid treatment plan, and if it is, you can move forward with the process in order to see if a direct stimulator will aid you in overcoming your pathologies once and for all.

If you wish to take control of your vagus nerve yourself, you can begin some of the techniques discussed within this book. Particularly for the yoga, breathing, and mindfulness techniques, you may choose to look into other books for more on how to trigger the desired states. You can learn several techniques to trigger mindfulness or more yoga poses that may help you feel better in no time.

No matter what, there is no real right answer on where to go from here. The best answer is the one that helps you lessen your own suffering. Whether you are currently suffering from anxiety, arthritis, epilepsy, or any other chronic illness or disorder that is causing you to be unhappy, what matters most is that you can trigger the happiness that you deserve, once and for all. With the help of the vagus nerve, you should be able to achieve that result with ease.

Lastly, if you felt that this book was beneficial to you in any way, if you learned even one useful thing, feedback is always greatly appreciated. Please do not hesitate to return to Amazon and leave a review for this book! Thank you for embarking on this journey, and good luck in your future endeavors!

www.ingramcontent.com/pod-product-compliance
Lightning Source LLC
Chambersburg PA
CBHW060332030426
42336CB00011B/1311